Praise for

What Makes You Tick?
A New Paradigm for Neuroscience

"Dr. Verschuuren is a refreshing voice in this misguided, half-truthed neuro world we live in today. There is as much, if not more, to learn about what the brain *isn't* than what it is and getting these illusions straight will help us all be able to live in truth.

Kudos to Dr. Verschuuren to have such a courageous voice...."

Kevin J. Fleming, Ph.D.
Founder
Grey Matters International, Inc.

"*What Makes You Tick* is a helpful guide on the self and its brain. It brings together a number of related themes, making complicated concepts understandable and exposing the faulty thinking found in scientific reductionism.

Verschuuren's book serves as an important reminder about what is at stake in the mind-brain discussion."

Paul Copan
Professor and Pledger Family Chair of Philosophy and Ethics
Palm Beach Atlantic University
West Palm Beach, Florida

"...there are few earthly realities as complex, or as fascinating...as the human brain. Recognizing this complexity, Dr. Verschuuren brings together ideas from philosophy, physics, genetics, and neuroscience to suggest a new paradigm for neuroscience.

While the intra-disciplinary ideas will be subject to the criticism from each of these fields, Verschuuren has succeeded indirectly in raising anew the perennial question of how a university should be constructed to allow for interdisciplinarity. The brainy dialogue of disciplines undertaken here provokes the further question of what makes our universities tick."

Richard Schenk OP
President of the Catholic University of Eichstaett-Ingolstadt

This welcome book brings neuroscience and metaphysics together in a way that does not seek so much to "solve" the mind-brain problem as to manifest the mystery of the human person as both physical and spiritual. From that perspective it is able to unmask the pseudo-dilemmas of scientism and the false "solutions" of materialism and dualism.

Maintaining the unity of the human person by a judicious use of the philosophy of Aristotle and Thomas Aquinas, it provides a way, in Verschuuren's astute phrase, for "telling the mental and physical apart without setting them apart."

Michael J. Dodds, O.P.
Professor of Philosophy and Theology
Dominican School of Philosophy & Theology
at the Graduate Theological Union
Berkeley, California

"This important book will compel psychiatrists, psychologists and others who work with patients within the neuroscience paradigm to reconsider some of the assumptions that drive their work while simultaneously encouraging clergy and pastoral counselors who do not traditionally work within that paradigm to engage with it."

John R.Siberski, M.D., S.J.
Associate Professor of Psychiatry
Georgetown University Medical School

What Makes You Tick?

A
NEW
PARADIGM
FOR
NEUROSCIENCE

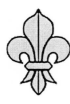

By: Gerard M. Verschuurren

Solas Press
Antioch
2012

Copyright © 2012 Gerard Verschuuren

Published by:
SOLAS Press
4627 Shetland Way
Antioch CA 94531
USA
www.solaspress.com

Library of Congress Cataloging-in-Publication Data

Verschuuren, G. M. N. (Geert M. N.)

What makes you tick? : a new paradigm for neuroscience / Gerard Verschuuren.

p. cm.

Includes bibliographical references and index.

Summary: "The book explores scientific determinism and its relation to the nature of material and nonmaterial entities. It proposes a new approach to benefit neuroscience in dealing with the human mind and mental concepts"-- Provided by publisher.

ISBN 978-1-893426-04-7

1. Cognitive neuroscience. 2. Thought and thinking. I. Title.

QP360.5.V475 2012

612.8'233--dc23

2012021275

Acknowledgements

I wish to first express my gratitude to the many persons, who must be nameless, who steered and corrected me in the process of preparation for this book. They make me realize that originality often consists in the capacity of forgetting about your sources. I particularly want to mention Francisco Ayala of the University of California at Irvine, the late John Huizinga of Utrecht University Medical School in the Netherlands, Peter Kreeft of Boston College, Kenneth R. Miller of Brown University, Wim J. Van Der Steen of Free University in Amsterdam, and the late Cornelius Van Peursen of Leiden University in the Netherlands whose critical scholarship influenced my ideas. I also thank Dominic Colvert, my editor at Solas Press, for his generous assistance and many key suggestions for the development of the manuscript. Obviously, they are not responsible for the outcome; if there are errors they are entirely my doing.

And—as with all my books in English—I could not have written this book without the unwavering and loving support of my wife, Trudy. I also want to specifically mention the great and helpful comments of our grandson Thomas J. Kelley, who is a senior at Westfield College, Massachusetts.

Foreword

When I was beginning my career as a neurosurgeon, my wife and I vacationed in Hudson, Wisconsin. Upon signing the register where we were staying in a grand old antebellum mansion we learned, it just so happened, that the house had been the boyhood home of the famous neurosurgeon, Dr. Wilder Penfield. As a fledgling resident neurosurgeon, I had used surgical tools named for Penfield but knew little about him—who he was and why he was so important to the field of neurosurgery.

Penfield graduated from high school in Hudson and matriculated to Princeton University. After a stellar academic career, he became a Rhodes Scholar in 1913 and traveled to Oxford, England; there he met Sir Charles Sherrington. Sherrington was a Nobel laureate and president of the Royal Society in the early 1920s; and at that time was described as the world's foremost neurophysiologist. I soon learned that it was Sherrington who made Penfield realize that the nervous system was the "undiscovered country"—the unexplored field in which the mystery of the mind of man might some day be explained. The main reason I had chosen neurosurgery as a career was the vast "undiscovered country" that was the brain—my interest was piqued!

Penfield in his time studied with the best minds in the field of neuroscience. Surmising that by seeing the brain in action he could contribute much to our knowledge of how the brain worked, he became a neurophysiologist and surgeon. In human patients under local anesthesia, he was able to observe directly the living brain and map out the responses to electrical stimulation. While treating patients suffering from epileptic seizures, he would surgically expose parts of the brain and electrically stimulate brain tissue in fully conscious patients. As an electrode was moved across the cerebral cortex, he was often able to locate the area of damaged brain tissue causing the epilepsy, remove it, and cure the epilepsy.

Penfield also found that stimulating certain parts of the brain could elicit vivid memories, songs, smells, movements, and emotions. Patients were regularly able to meticulously describe very remote events in great detail, while at the same time being fully conscious of the surgeon's activity. Each time he would stimulate an area again, the memory or song would return. In a film, Penfield discusses stimulating a woman's brain where she recalled a very specific tune, and she recounts it on the same film—how magnificent! Penfield marveled at the memories evoked by electrical stimulation, they were like recorded television programs being replayed in the mind of the patient—programs so vivid that patients could even smell coffee and hear sounds. Yet the patients were always fully conscious, aware of being in surgery, and aware that these were triggered memories. He termed this *double consciousness.*

After an immensely successful neurosurgical career during which he was at one time called "the greatest living Canadian," Penfield took up a second career in 1960. In this, much like his one-time mentor Sir Charles Sherrington, he devoted the final years of his life to unraveling the mysteries of the mind. Given the advances in neurosurgery and neuroscience the question naturally arose whether someday we would find—as the philosopher Rene Descartes had contemplated—that the "seat of the soul" would be found somewhere in the gray or white matter of the cerebral substance? Penfield describes his original premise that with time the mind will be completely explained by physics, chemistry and the neuronal circuitry. But gradually, and through his experience with his patients his thinking evolved:

> Throughout my own scientific career I, like the other scientists, have struggled to prove that the brain accounts for the mind. But now, perhaps, the time has come when we may profitably consider the evidence as it stands, and ask the question: "Do brain mechanisms account for the mind?" Can the mind be explained by what is now known about the brain? If not, which is the more reasonable of the two possible hypotheses: that man's being is based on one element, or on two?[1]

---

[1] Wilder Penfield, *The Mystery of the Mind, A Critical Study of Consciousness and the Human Brain* (Princeton, N.J.: Princeton University Press, 1975), xiii.

Penfield likening the brain to a computer, he did not believe that the man *was* a computer, rather, that he *had* a computer—and that this computer has a programmer. He said, "There is a switchboard operator as well as a switchboard."

Once he asked his patient to try and resist the movement of the patient's left arm that he was about to make move by stimulating the motor cortex in the right hemisphere of the brain. The patient grabbed his left arm with his right hand, attempting to restrict the movement that was to be induced by surgeons' stimulation of the right brain. Thus the left hemisphere was telling the right hand to restrict the movement of the left arm being forced to move by the stimulation of the right hemisphere. As Penfield said, "Behind the brain action of one hemisphere was the patient's *mind*. Behind the action of the other hemisphere was the electrode."

Sir Charles Sherrington, who retired in 1936, did not have the benefit of studying the brain in awake, living, breathing, conscious beings who could describe their experiences. After his lifetime in studying neurophysiology in monkeys, dogs, cats, and other animals, he became a philosopher and penned *Man on His Nature*—a series of lectures delivered on his concepts of the mind-brain relationship.[2] Five days before he died, he said to one of his star pupils, Sir John Eccles, "For me now, the only reality is the *human soul*"[3]

Sir John Eccles, as a young man studying physiology, was not satisfied with the scientific explanations of the mind-brain interaction, and this influenced his decision to become a neuroscientist. After a brilliant career as a neuroscientist, during which he was honored with the 1963 Nobel Prize in medicine and physiology, Eccles retired in 1975 to devote himself, like Sherrington, to the study of the mind-brain problem. He published

---

[2] See Charles Scott Sherrington, *Man on his Nature*, 2nd ed. (Cambridge, Eng: University Press, 1951).

[3] John C. Eccles, *Facing Reality: Philosophical Adventures of a Brain Scientist* (London: Longman; New York: Springer-Verlag, Heidelberg Science Library, 1970), 174.

no less than seven books about the mind-brain interaction, culminating in his 1994 work *How the Self Controls its Brain.*[4]

What was it that prompted these eminent neuroscientists to end their brilliant careers seeking to explain the relationship of the mind to the brain? Why were they so unsatisfied with the purely scientific explanations of the mind? Why did they raise the question—can and does the mind exist independent of the brain? In this book Dr. Gerard Verschuuren explores a new paradigm to explain the mind-brain interface. He is, with his background as a human geneticist and his study of the philosophy of science, uniquely qualified to discuss these concepts. He is at once conversant in the language of the Darwinist and the Theologian, and the dualist and the physicalist. His experience as a teacher of biology, human genetics, statistics, philosophy, and logic is evident in the exceptionally readable prose that illumines what is often a very difficult topic to understand.

The new paradigm that Verschuuren proposes will require an innovative way of thinking among those who are not used to thinking outside the box. Rather than the reductionist, materialistic approach of neuroscience today, Verschuuren asks that we consider a paradigm that does not rely exclusively on biological substrata and physics. Far from dismissing science and physics, he demonstrates how any cogent theory of mind must also include metaphysical constructs. As Eccles noted:

> The more we discover about the brain, the more clearly do we distinguish between the brain events and the mental phenomena, and the more wonderful do both the brain events and the mental phenomena become. Promissory materialism is simply a religious belief held by dogmatic materialists...who often confuse their religion with their science.[5]

Like Penfield, I am fortunate to have the opportunity to work on a daily basis with the magnificent organ that houses the mind.

---

[4] John C. Eccles, *How the Self Controls its Brain* (Berlin: Springer-Verlag, 1994).

[5] John C. Eccles and Daniel N. Robinson, *The Wonder of Being Human: Our Brain and Our Mind* (Boston: New Science Library, 1984), 36.

In this book Verschuuren has given *my* brain much to contemplate as I peer into the operating microscope, and has helped my mind comprehend why I am so intrigued with the opportunity to continue to study the brain.

— Paul J. Camarata, M.D., FACS
Chairman, Department of Neurosurgery
University of Kansas School of Medicine

Contents

Preface

The study of the human brain has a venerable and inspiring history. Opening the skull—trepanation—has been performed since prehistoric times. When surgeons of the modern era finally attempted to penetrate deeper into the interior of the human body, into the abdominal and thoracic cavities, they opened up a world that had been considered untouchable for centuries. Then new discoveries emboldened surgery to extend its domain to the human brain. If men of the Stone Age had without anesthesia or antisepsis perfected the technique of trepanation, we, with our modern achievements, should surely be able to perform such operations successfully and thus open the inner chambers of cerebral powers and combat diseases.

But even to this day there is an extraordinary thrill about the idea of brain surgery. For is not the brain still to some extent, as it was in prehistory, the most mysterious part of our bodies; the apparently unfathomable and inviolable center of all our feeling, thinking, and acting—perhaps of our souls?

Brain research may have started slowly but it has speeded up dramatically. The advancements of brain research are mind-boggling, and many promises are still awaiting us. In the same way that DNA research experienced a rapid acceleration in the late twentieth century, something similar is now happening in the world of brain research. Because I was brought up in a world of science, "brain-washed" by scientists during my studies in biology and human genetics, surrounded by scientists when I became involved with research and teaching, I have learned to greatly value these achievements.

Isn't it amazing how we seem to have demystified this center of all our feeling, thinking, acting, and perhaps of our souls? What has helped tremendously is the fact that we treat the human body, including its brain, as some kind of contraption that runs and ticks with clockwork precision that can be manipulated once we know its mechanisms. We can use chemicals to interfere with its processes. We can even use animals to learn more about brain mechanisms; since it is supposed we are all alike—"cut from the same cloth." As a result, we know more and more about what makes us "tick." That, I believe, is the end result of all these new developments in neuroscience. I want to be the last one to deny the tremendous value of these discoveries; and yet there is something missing in this picture.

What is missing in the picture of science, and of neuroscience in particular, that I have painted? Science is certainly an imposing enterprise, but it cannot account for all that needs to be accounted for. Some think that *all* our questions have scientific answers phrased in terms of particles, quantities, and equations. To best characterize this attitude I will borrow an image from the late psychologist Abraham Maslow: "If you only have a hammer, every problem begins to look like a nail." The current discoveries are what the "scientific hammer" has achieved. The astonishing successes of science have not been gained by answering every kind of question but precisely by refusing to do so.

If human beings were, as some have suggested, nothing but a string of DNA or a pack of neurons, they would be pretty fragile creatures; and even this very claim would be worth nothing more than the DNA and the neurons that supposedly produced that claim. To argue differently amounts to *scientism*. The ideology of scientism would shackle us in a physical, material world. However, making the claim that there is only physical matter implies that this very claim does not and cannot exist because claims are essentially not physical. And if such a non-physical claim does exist there must be more than physical matter in this universe. When we deny the existence of things immaterial, we also deny the existence of our own immaterial denial—as well as all our scientific claims. *Scientism steps outside scientific territory to claim that there is nothing outside scientific territory.* It declares everything outside science as an unacceptable form of metaphysics, without realizing that those who reject metaphysics are actually practicing their own version of metaphysics. Metaphysics may be a "dirty word" to some, but we are surrounded by it—like it or not.

In this book I make a claim for something that is more than physics—and that is where we inevitably enter the territory of metaphysics. This book takes you from the all too familiar, rock-solid world of molecules, genes, cells, and neurons to a world beyond the world of physics. In other words, I take neuro-*science* seriously, but without turning it into neuro-*mania*. As a matter of fact, there is much more, as Shakespeare's Hamlet put it, "than dreamt of in your philosophy."

I invite you to follow me on this journey into the "Grand Beyond." When I wrote the book, I had in mind a semi-serious book—serious in content, but light in style and format, profound but not heavy, engaging but not strenuous. I believe I came up with a book that gives you food for thought—a thoughtful book that includes mind and spirit.

In the first three chapters, I argue that it is not molecules, DNA, or not even neurons that make you "tick." The chapters after that address some thought provoking issues: is the "mind" just a matter of "matter," or is there something like "mind over matter"? What makes the mind different from the brain, and from everything that comes with the brain—cells, genes, DNA, molecules? Are we really just walking brains? Are we really nothing but "a vast assembly of nerve cells and their associated molecules," as Francis Crick once announced in his book *The Astonishing Hypothesis*? My competing hypothesis states that the brain is different from the mind, and that mind research is different from brain research, and that brain surgeons are not mind surgeons. This amounts to telling the mental and the physical apart, yet without setting them apart.

This approach obviously stands in sharp contrast with the current paradigm used in neuroscience. The current paradigm of neuroscience—which I will now call the "old" paradigm—is too materialistic, too deterministic, and too reductionistic to do justice to the unique position of human beings in this world. Neuroscience now calls for a more comprehensive, more inclusive paradigm, which I hope to offer you in the last two chapters.

At the end of some chapters, you will find something that I call an intermission. You can skip them or devour them depending on your appetite. Bon appétit

WHAT MAKES YOU TICK?
A NEW PARADIGM FOR NEUROSCIENCE

Chapter 1

Clockwork

In my grandparents' house there was a huge grandfather clock. As a kid I used to stand in front of it, wondering what made it tick. Nowadays I have an idea: an intricate network of cogs and wheels makes it work with the precision of clockwork. But I also know that this clock will stop working if the cascade of causes was not set into motion by another cause—someone winding up the spring. But no matter how you look at it, what we have here is one thing setting another thing in motion. That is how our world too seems to work—as a chain of events following one after another according to the law of cause and effect.

Why would you and I be in any way an exception? Even our own bodies seem to be in the grip of some rigid clockwork mechanism. If we do not eat, we die. If there is no oxygen, we gasp for breath. If we drink too much alcohol, our brains are affected. If we imbibe poison, death sets in. Like it or not, we are in the grip of some form of determinism; every cause has an inevitable and inescapable effect. So must it be that those causes make *you* tick?

Indeed, determinism sounds very attractive. It allows us, for instance, to forecast the weather. Today's weather depends on what happened yesterday, and so will tomorrow's weather depend on today's. If meteorologists give you a faulty forecast they can always blame something—the inaccuracy of the data, the complexity of the calculations, and so on—but never will they give up the idea of determinism. Science would not be possible if it did not assume that like causes have like effects and that the future depends on the past. The orderliness of this universe is a prerequisite for science. However, if like causes always produce like effects, then the past appears to fully determine the future. Does that not sound compelling? It seems there is no way out: we end up with the doctrine of complete causal determinism, which the French astronomer Pierre Simon Laplace worded emphatically as follows: "We may regard the present state of the universe as the effect of its past and as the cause of its future."[1]

Even Hollywood dealt with this issue in the 1944 movie *It Happened Tomorrow*. It portrayed a man, Lawrence Stevens, mysteriously receiving the newspaper of the next day. This interesting feature enabled Stevens to be prepared for what was ahead of him, including an assault on his life, which he tried, of course, to escape, but in vain. Natural laws could be likened to the newspapers of the days ahead of us. If the doctrine of complete determinism were true, then our universe would run like clockwork, with no capacity for caprice or free choice. The future would be completely determined by the past.

I said, "*If* the doctrine of complete determinism were true..." Indeed, I consider determinism to be a doctrine, not a matter of fact. And mind you, doctrines may not be true! What then could be wrong with determinism?

Some think determinism is a mere illusion, because the notion of causality is supposed to be only a human artifact. Those who claim this tend to walk in the footsteps of the Scottish philosopher David Hume. Indeed, Hume was one of the first *skeptic* philosophers, who put into question the very idea of objective truth—which would also include the truth of causality and determinism. In order to do so, he uses the famous example of a billiard ball moving in a straight line toward another ball.[2] There are several possibilities: the first ball bounces back, with the second ball remaining at rest; the first ball stops and the second ball moves; or the first ball jumps over the second, and so on. There is no reason to conclude any of these possibilities over the others. Only through previous observation can it be predicted what will actually happen with the balls. All we observe is that the motion of the first billiard ball is followed by the motion of the second ball: we cannot observe the act of *causation*. Nor does the mind perceive the workings of cause and effect; otherwise we could determine what effects would follow from causes without ever having to rely on observation. Furthermore, we do not actually experience

---

[1] Pierre Simon Laplace (1749–1827), *A Philosophical Essay on Probabilities*, 6th edition, trans. into English from the original French by F. W. Truscott and F. L. Emory (New York: Dover Publications, 1951), 4.

[2] David Hume, *Enquiry Concerning Human Understanding*, Third Edition, ed. Peter Nidditch (Oxford: Oxford University Press, 1975), §4.1.

the necessary connection itself: we only infer it from the constant conjunction that we observe between two events.

No wonder Hume used this example, because at the time the billiard-ball model had become standard in explaining the nature of the universe—which is determinism in its full glory. In addition, the billiard-ball model stood for a kind of causal action that was thought to be evident, because the mechanism of this kind of action was supposedly clear and all-pervading. It was an example of "impulse," that is, of one body causing changes in another body by means of contact—by pushing it or striking it. "Impulse," John Locke once wrote, is "the only way which we can conceive Bodies operate in."[3] What Hume did, in contrast, was argue that this "mechanism" was really a kind of illusion produced by habit or custom. All such cases are supposedly nothing but constant conjunctions, and our perceptions of them never give us insight into the modus operandi of the connection. Causal connections turned out to be mere "metaphysical" inventions, based on an illusion.

What is wrong with Hume's analysis? Notice what is being affirmed here: that something metaphysical such as "causal connections" depends on what the imagination creates. Hume came to this view because he took causality as a relationship of *events*, assuming that "all events seem entirely loose and separate" and that "we can never observe any tie between them." As a consequence, causal connections in themselves are ultimately subjective phenomena in Hume's view. How different is this view of causality compared to the Aristotelian view: cause and effect is rooted in the identity of acting things. What a thing is, says Aristotle, will determine what it does. An acorn can become an oak tree, and not a catfish, because that is its nature. The actions an entity can take are determined by what that entity is. On this latter view, when one billiard ball strikes another, it sends it rolling because of the nature of the balls and their surroundings, not just antecedent events. When we know that billiard balls are solid and when we see one ball moving toward another, then certain effects are quite impossible. The moving ball cannot, for example, just pass through the second ball and come out the other side, continuing at the same speed; nor can the first ball stop at exactly the same place as the second ball; nor can one of the

---

[3] John Locke, *Essay Concerning Human Understanding*, viii, 11.

balls suddenly vanish, and so on. The qualities of the balls determine the kind of effect that the impulse of the first ball will have on the second.[4]

Moreover, the law of causality is an objective given: contrary to Hume's notion that causal connections ultimately depend on the input of human imagination, causality seen as a relationship between an entity and its own actions exists independently of our consciousness. If you see entities acting, you see causality. If Hume were right, the law of a daily sunrise is not "out there," but is merely a mental conception based on our habit of seeing the sun rise every morning. If natural laws were just mental habits, it would be hard to explain why bridges built in accordance with the proper physical laws and boundary conditions stand firm, whereas others collapse. Would competent engineers really have better mental habits than their inept colleagues? There has got to be more to it! G. K. Chesterton once "seriously joked" about a conspiracy of order in our world of regularity: "One elephant having a trunk was odd, but all elephants having trunks looked like a plot."[5] Well, science is in search of that plot.

In spite of contrary claims made by David Hume and his followers, we do have knowledge of an external world. Although we know the world through sensations or sense impressions, they are just the *media* that give us access to reality. The philosopher John Haldane put it well when he said:

> One only knows about cats and dogs through sensations, but they are not themselves sensations, any more than the players in a televised football game are color patterns on a flat screen.[6]

Knowledge does rest on sensation, but that doesn't mean it is confined to it. The Scholastics observed that there is nothing in the mind that was not first in the senses. What they meant is that what is immediately sensed—"qualities" or "impressions" in Hume's terminology, such as colors, sounds, and odors—are only the media

---

[4] See James Hill, "On Billiard Balls—Hume Against The Mechanists," *Richmond Journal of Philosophy*, 3 (2003): 22-26.

[5] G. K. Chesterton, *Orthodoxy* (New York: John Lane, 1908), 106-7.

[6] John Haldane, "Hume's Destructive Genius," *First Things*, 218 (2011): 23-25.

through which reality is discerned and understood, but we are not confined to those sensations.

If we were to follow Hume's philosophy, we would end up with what the physicist and historian of science Stanley Jaki calls, "bricks without mortar." He says about Hume's sensations:

> The bricks he used for construction were sensory impressions. Merely stacking bricks together never produces an edifice, let alone an edifice that is supposed to be the reasoned edifice of knowledge."[7]

Hume leaves us in a cognitive desert.

Curiously enough, Hume rejects metaphysical entities on metaphysical grounds. He reduces reality—that which *is*—to mere sensations. He certainly is not joined by giants of physics such as Max Planck and Albert Einstein, who both believed that physical laws describe a reality independent of ourselves, and that the theories of physics show not only how nature behaves, but why it behaves exactly as it does and not otherwise. We are dealing here with truth and reason, not sentiment and habit. So the bottom line is that there is still space left for determinism—there seems to be some kind of "law and order" in this universe. But how far does this form of determinism go?

I must admit that determinism may very well make sense within the general framework of science and within the models proposed and used by science. What do I mean by that? Science, including meteorology, always works with models. Scientific models are like maps—simplified versions of the original they represent or depict. Think of highway maps, railroad maps, vegetation maps, and so on. "Good" scientists are those able to demarcate their areas of investigation, able to limit themselves to factors that are relevant to their objects of investigation, and capable of eliminating from consideration any factors that might interfere with their research by keeping those that would interfere under strict control. Much of the genius of research workers lies in their selection of what is worth investigating so they can reduce their many questions to a manageable problem.

---

[7] Stanley Jaki, *The Road of Science and the Ways to God* (The University of Chicago Press, 1978), 103.

The Nobel laureate Peter Medawar described research as a real art—he called it "the art of the soluble."[8] Whatever is not yet soluble is not now a good object of investigation. Scientists are specialized in measuring and counting, but ironically, not everything that "counts" can be counted. No wonder most sciences have been successful, since they were able to create a test-tube-like shelter in a laboratory removed from the complexity of nature so that the various factors under investigation can be isolated and manipulated on an individual basis. Eventually, this leads to a "map" of what is going on in this world.

Maps are very useful only if we have the right map; a railroad map would be quite useless for motorists. Consequently, we end up with a variety of maps, each one made for a specific purpose and depicting a distinct aspect of the world: a meteorological map, a biological map, a chemical map, an economic map, and so on. These maps complement each other in describing and explaining disparate phenomena, which represent distinct aspects of the same world. But it is clear there is no "universal" map. Such an all-inclusive "map" would be the real world itself, and as complex as the real world. All scientific maps and models are just abstract representations of the original world—and for that matter, very limited replicas. So scientific maps and models are not to be confused with the real phenomena they represent. The philosopher Gilbert Ryle phrased this idea in his own terminology:

> As the painter in oils on one side of the mountain and the painter in water-colors on the other side of the mountain produce very different pictures, which may still be excellent pictures of the same mountain, so the nuclear physicist, the theologian, the historian, the lyric poet and the man in the street produce very different, yet compatible and even complementary pictures of one and the same "world."[9]

What does all of this have to do with our issue of determinism? Well, the doctrine of determinism detaches natural laws and chains of cause-and-effect from their scientific models and then applies them beyond their range to the world in its entirety. However, whenever

---

[8] P. B. Medawar, *The Art of the Soluble* (New York: Barnes and Noble, 1967).

[9] Gilbert Ryle, "The World of Science and the Everyday World," *Dilemmas* (Cambridge University Press, 1960, paperback), 68 - 81.

we apply certain statements to "everything," we might run into contradictions. What we have here is, in essence, the problem of so-called self-reference. This problem is known from the famous Liar Paradox: Epimenides, a Cretan, says, "All Cretans are liars." Is Epimenides telling the truth or not? If he is, he is not; if he is not, he is. The philosopher Bertrand Russell[10] rephrased this paradox in more general terms: Let R be the set of all the sets which do not contain themselves as an element. Does R then belong to that set? Is the set of all sets which are not members of themselves also a member of itself? If it is, then it is not. If it is not, then it is. Whatever answer we choose, we are led into contradiction.

From this, Russell drew the conclusion that there is no set of *all* sets, for the notion of a set of all sets which includes itself as a member generates paradoxes. Applied to our case, this would mean that the doctrine of complete determinism is a self-defeating proposition, because it leads to contradictions. Any scientific claim about determinism is necessarily bound to the specific setting of a specific model and does not automatically hold for situations outside that model, let alone for itself. In other words, determinism is not an all-pervasive phenomenon, because it would be valid only within the setting of a model. In that specific sense, determinism cannot claim *universal* validity for *local* successes. The astonishing successes of science have not been gained by answering every kind of question, but precisely by refusing to do so.

So we have a problem here. Determinism in its all-pervasive version is self-defeating—if it is true, it becomes false. If I say that all human beings are liars, then the very statement I am making as a human being must be a lie too. Similarly, when determinists want to include everything in the universe, it must include the doctrine of determinism as well. This makes this very doctrine also the result of an inescapable chain of causes and effects. In other words, trying to persuade others of complete determinism would be a useless enterprise, since convictions are supposedly predetermined anyway. Of course, we could immunize the doctrine of determinism by claiming that it cannot refer to itself. But that is a desperate strategy, for if we let in one statement that is not predetermined, many others

---

[10] Bertrand Russell, "Logic and Knowledge," *American Journal of Mathematics*, Vol. 30 (1908): 222-262.

may follow. So I would suggest limiting its validity to a smaller domain—for instance, the domain of science and its models.

That takes us to another reason for questioning the doctrine of determinism—a reason based on common sense and intuition. When we watch a game on the golf course or on the pool table, we see balls following precisely determined courses of cause and effect; they follow physical laws and are subject to well-known rules. But there is one element that does not seem to fit in this predetermined picture— the players of the game themselves. I am deliberately using the same example as David Hume did, but this time to show that there are entities and factors active on the pool table that Hume seemed to be blind to. I would say to him that there is the David Hume who wants to be the philosopher and the David Hume who plays billiards. Using his own words, "Be a philosopher; but amidst all your philosophy, be still a man."[11]

As we all know, the direction of something like a billiard ball on the pool table or a golf ball on the golf course is ruled not only by physical laws but also by human intentions—by players who have a certain goal in mind. These players somehow fall outside the realm of the model of physics; they can steer the course of the laws of nature. The players are similar to engineers who manipulate nature for technological reasons.

Of course, you could object here and argue that these players and engineers are also part of a completely deterministic system—with all their actions predetermined like clockwork—but that requires a lot of imagination. As the Nobel-laureate and physicist Arthur Holly Compton has said:

> If the laws of physics ever should come to contradict my conviction that I can move my little finger at will, then all the laws of physics should be revised and reformulated.[12]

Even in a world ruled by the law of cause and effect, there is also our own ability to be the cause of events.

---

[11] David Hume, *Enquiry*, Section 1, 9.

[12] Arthur Holly Compton, et al., *Man's Destiny in Eternity. (A Book from a Symposium. The Garvin Lectures)* (Boston: Beacon Press, 1949). Note that Compton has the distinction of being the discoverer of the Compton Effect.

That takes us to a third problem with determinism. An all-pervasive determinist doctrine wants me to *believe* that everything is predetermined. But how could it *make* me believe so, for wouldn't my beliefs be as predestined as anything else in life? In other words, people who defend complete determinism—let us call them determinists—want me to *choose* their conviction that human beings *cannot* choose. I would say to them, "Predict my behavior and I will do otherwise." Of course, the determinists may counter that this would be predictable as well had they been given "enough" information. To which I would respond that it is very hard to make predictions, in particular when the future is concerned!

In short, thinking that we "tick" like a clock cannot be proved; although it can be a conviction that some people have despite evidence to the contrary. I conclude that the answer to the question featured in the title of this book —*What Makes You Tick?*—cannot be found in a simple "clockwork" mechanism or in cascades of physical causes and effects only. Do our lives really unwind like grandfather clocks, with the same precise course and the same fixed outcome? Determinism is part of the answer, but there is certainly more to it. What then could that "more" be?

Intermission 1A

A Technical Defeat of Determinism

It will be worthwhile to mention something about Turing Machines in the context of determinism. Without going into technical details, a Turing Machine is a device that manipulates symbols on a strip of tape. The Turing Machine is not intended to be a practical computing technology, but rather to be a hypothetical device representing a computing machine. What is important to our discussion is the fact that Turing Machines help computer scientists understand the limits of mechanical computation.

One of the things Alan Turing proved with his computational-machine model is "that there can be no general process or algorithm for determining whether a given formula U of the functional calculus K is provable. So that there can not be a machine that supplied with any one U of these formulae will eventually say whether U is provable."[1] In a second proof, Turing shows that if one asks for a general procedure to show: "Does this machine ever print zero?" the question is "undecidable."

In a similar vein, I would like to point to a classic technique for proving that a system is deficient by demonstrating that it creates contradictions or inconsistencies. The philosopher and physicist Karl Popper used this technique to show that the notion of overall determinism is inherently wrong.[2] He achieved his point by first supposing that we have a huge computer that can predict the future based on data regarding all initial conditions and all the laws needed to derive effects from causes. The machine gives answers by turning a lamp on in case of "no" and off in case of "yes." Now we feed the data and ask the computer to predict whether the lamp will be on or off

---

[1] Alan Turing (1912–1954),"On Computable Numbers, With an Application to the Entscheidungsproblem," *The Undecidable* , ed.,Martin Davis, (Hewlett, NY: Raven Press, 1965): 145.

[2] See Karl Popper, *Conjectures and Refutations: The Growth of Scientific Knowledge* (London: Routledge, 1963).

after ninety-nine years. After going through numerous calculations, the computer predicts that the lamp will be *on* by actually switching the lamp *off* (or reversed)—which makes either prediction wrong. This result demonstrates that there is something wrong with the presuppositions of complete determinism.

Here are numerous possible arguments why determinism may be wrong: not all necessary data and/or laws can be specified; prediction is inherently different from explanation; a computer with enough computational power does not exist; prediction-before-the-fact always takes so much time that it becomes explanation-after-the-fact; or determinism is just not an all-pervasive phenomenon. Personally, I favor the argument that determinism is not an all-pervasive phenomenon. It is true only in limited, demarcated areas that leave space for what is called "free will."

However, there seems to be some recent experimental evidence that free will is just an illusion. I am referring here to Benjamin Libet's famous experiments, which appear to demonstrate that so-called conscious decisions are already settled before we become aware of them. He asked his experimental subjects to move one hand at an arbitrary moment decided by them, and to report when the decision was made, which was timed by noticing the position of a dot circling a clock face at the moment of decision. In the meantime, the electrical activity of their brains was monitored. Earlier research had already indicated that consciously chosen actions are preceded by a pattern of activity known as a Readiness Potential (RP). RP is a measurable electrical change in the brain that precedes an act that we choose to make, which would make RP a good marker for a decision. Well, it turned out that the reported time of each decision was always a short period (some tenths of a second) *after* the RP appeared. This outcome seems to prove that the supposedly conscious decisions are actually determined unconsciously beforehand.

If the decision to move is really made half a second before we are consciously aware of having decided, how could our conscious thoughts have determined what the decision was? Isn't that the end of the free will debate? I have my doubts! There are many problems with this experiment. I won't go into all the details, but just raise a few pertinent questions.

First, one might argue that these experiments are based more on training than on conscious intervention. The experiment could well be measuring just a trained reaction time. Perhaps simple decisions like pressing a button do not require much mental intervention by reasoning or other mental considerations. Experiments such as these do not seem to represent normal decision-making for we do not typically make random decisions at a random moment of our choosing. Benjamin Libet asked his subjects to merely "let the urge [to move] appear on its own at any time without any pre-planning or concentration on when to act."[3] However, one cannot passively wait for an urge to occur while at the same time being the one who is consciously bringing it about.

On another level of interpretation, we should question whether the RP really is a signal that a decision has been made. Since the occurrence of an RP in the brain indicated that a movement was coming along just afterward, it was taken as a neurological sign that the decision to move had been made. However, when I make a decision about my house mortgage, does an RP appear, or is it only wrist movements that cause RPs? In these experiments, the experimental subjects were required to get into a frame of mind where they were ready to make a decision at any moment. Perhaps the RP merely signals a quickening of attention, rather than a moment of decision? Further research by Trevena and Miller that not only included situations when there was movement but also situations when the subject decided not to move indicates that the same kind of RP appeared whether or not the subject pressed a key— thus making the RP rather an indication of some general kind of attention or preparation for a decision.[4] The authors concluded "that Libet's results do not provide evidence that voluntary movements are initiated unconsciously."[5]

---

[3] B. Libet, E. W. Wright, C. A. Gleason, "Readiness potentials preceding unrestricted spontaneous pre-planned voluntary acts," *Electroencephalographic and Clinical Neurophysiology*, 54 (1983): 322–325.

[4] J. A. Trevena and J. Miller, "Cortical movement preparation before and after a conscious decision to move," *Consciousness and Cognition*, 11 (2002): 162–190.

[5] J. A. Trevena and J. Miller, "Brain preparation before a voluntary action: Evidence against unconscious movement initiation", *Consciousness and Cognition*, 19 (2010): 447–456.

From the logic of the experimental situation you know that whenever you have decided to do something the decision has, by definition, already been made. In other words, the RP demonstrates that the expected brain activity always occurs *before* a decision but does not reveal the *result* of the decision. Any test that shows a delay just shows that subjects can indeed delay an action until after they have confirmed that they are conscious of the decision to act. How could we consider ourselves responsible for decisions we were not even aware of until after they had been made?

One could also argue that these experiments involve at least *two* mental reporting processes: one having to do with the occurrence of the decision, and the other having to do with the state of the clock, which makes it hard to establish simultaneity. Those are in fact two different levels of awareness. It is highly possible that we need a certain amount of time just in order to report the awareness to ourselves. Being aware of the decision one has made is one thing, and being aware of that awareness is another—which might require more time to develop. The delay between decision and awareness does not mean the decision was not ours, any more than the short delay before we hear our own voice means we didn't intend what we said.

Considering the human organism, there is reason to question whether the brain is the "agent" of consciousness. Perhaps it is not the "agent" of consciousness, but rather the "instrument" of consciousness. If that is the case, the brain could very well be receiving instructions from elsewhere to execute choices. Part of these instructions could be stored somewhere in memory, but only *after* the instructions have been executed. We will discuss this issue much more extensively in the chapters to come.

Last but not least, the only evidence about what conscious experiences are like comes from first-person sources, from the very consciousness of an experimental subject. All reports of my mental activity come via the reporting entity, that is, "I myself." This fact is often overlooked, but it has enormous consequences: consciousness must be something more than mere neuronal activity. In order for us to make the connection between inner mental states and outer neural states, we necessarily depend on information that only the "brain-owner" can provide. We will revisit the question of inner mental states and outer neural states later.

In short, the above experiments are often explained from a deterministic viewpoint but can be explained from a non-deterministic perspective as well. Their outcome is very ambiguous.

Intermission 1B

The Debate on Determinism in Physics

There have always been, and undoubtedly always will be, scientists who think that the *metaphysical* presuppositions of order, causality, and functionality in this universe are mere scientific, empirical findings open to regular falsification—in ignorance of the fact that falsification would not work without the assumption of some underlying order. Recently, for instance, many scientists developed a new interest in chaos and chaotic systems, as if these could falsify the existence of order.

It is true that some natural systems can be described only by non-linear mathematical equations with such complex solutions that we cannot exactly predict what the system will do in the near future. Or to take another example, our measurements of all the initial conditions of a particular system (in, for example, meteorology) may be too numerous and/or too inaccurate to predict exactly what the outcome would be. However, this isn't really chaos, but only appears to be chaos. As a matter of fact, we are looking for the very order behind these seemingly chaotic phenomena. When the weather forecast is off the mark, does that mean the weather is unpredictable? No, of course it is not; we just do not know enough. And let us not forget that statistics—the science of randomness par excellence—is in itself a very orderly enterprise.

No wonder there was a passionate discussion in quantum physics between Albert Einstein and Niels Bohr. According to Heisenberg's principle of uncertainty or indeterminacy, it is impossible to determine simultaneously the values of position and momentum, or of energy and time, with any great degree of certainty; the more precisely one property is known, the less precisely can the other be known. The question, though, is how to interpret this phenomenon. In Bohr's interpretation, which is called the "principle of complementarity," these values are in essence undetermined until we measure one of them. Light, for example, behaves either as a wave or as a stream of particles, depending on our experimental setup, but we can never see both at the same time.

What Bohr's interpretation entails is that the role of the observer is crucial in the measurement; the measurement of position would necessarily disturb a particle's momentum, and vice versa. As a result, it is assumed that these quantities have no precise values, so the behavior of atoms and electrons can no longer be predicted until measured. Albert Einstein, on the other hand, always detested Bohr's interpretation. An electron's spin, for instance, only appears undefined, he said, because some variables are still hidden and unknown. If this stand is correct, uncertainty would be located not in the real world but in our knowledge of the real world.

As a philosopher of science, I tend to side with Einstein, whose philosophical qualifications would surpass those of Bohr. I must admit, though, that Bohr had a well managed public relations campaign for his interpretation and developed a powerful school of adherents—who included Heisenberg. Nevertheless, I prefer to join such giants of physics as Einstein, Max Planck, David Bohm, and Erwin Schrödinger, who have always maintained that natural laws describe a reality independent of ourselves, whereas Bohr's interpretation means that we have lost contact with reality and causality, because we are supposedly dealing with mere appearances, such as Geiger counts. A Humean solution!

Isn't it ironic how Bohr and his Copenhagen school try to give us a *causal* explanation of the alleged fact that *causal* explanations are impossible in their view? They think that we *do* not know because we *cannot* know. Besides, I would argue that it is logically impossible to prove that something has no cause. Causality can never be conclusively defeated by experiments, since causality is the metaphysical foundation of experiments. No wonder that Einstein spent the last four decades of his life in a quest to restore order to physics. He realized that order does not come from science but actually enables science.

Come what may, the indeterminacy debate is still very alive in physics at the present time, and is apparently...well, indeterminate. So how then can complete determinism be averted? Would indeterminacy in the quantum world offer us a solution? I do not think so. Bohr's and Heisenberg's interpretations posit that an electron's spin is undetermined until we measure it, but this is based on the assumption that the experimenter is free to decide on what is going to be measured, and when—otherwise it would have been determined ahead of time when the measurement is bound to occur and what its outcome then must be. So this interpretation assumes human freedom, but does not explain or produce it. And besides, it would be a long stretch to reason from physical indeterminacy to human freedom, for as we will see later, they occur at very different levels. I would say we need a better solution. I trust I have one for you in the upcoming chapters.

Chapter 2

A DNA Blueprint

Don't you agree that we are living in an exciting era? Science is making progress in leaps and bounds, sometimes even in giant leaps. Without science, the E of $E=mc^2$ would still equal E. And think of all the developments that molecular biology has achieved in a relatively short period of time since the discovery of DNA in 1953. Now that the Human Genome Project is finished, some believe we know all there is to be known about human beings. No wonder one of the DNA pioneers said he could compute the entire organism if he were given its DNA sequence and a large enough computer.[1] That organism could be you! Apparently DNA is the new candidate for what makes you tick.

This overconfident attitude has been very contagious. Many people think that DNA holds the script for a person's entire life, so they would like to know their "personal genomics." The science journal *Nature* listed "Personal Genomics Goes Mainstream" as a top news story of 2008. The clockwork mantra has been revitalized, albeit more refined, by going into the molecular details of our "destiny." The new genomics has now become our new crystal ball.

What do we know about DNA? Before Mendel, differences in temperament, talents, social status, wealth, and power were all believed to reside "in the blood."[2] With the rise of Mendelian genetics, genes were substituted for blood in the explanations. People differ in ABO blood types, for instance, because they carry a gene that can have different variants, called alleles; two of those determine the blood type they have. Doesn't this sound like a new form of determinism?

---

[1] This claim was made at a symposium in commemoration of the 100th anniversary of the death of Charles Darwin, by one of the founders of the molecular biology of the gene.

[2] Gregor Johann Mendel (1822–1884), an Austrian scientist and Augustinian friar. He gained posthumous fame as the founder of the new science of genetics.

Let us find out whether it holds. Some genes do indeed work in one single step. There is, for instance, a gene that produces, in one step, the enzyme tyrosinase, which creates the dark skin pigment melanin. This gene can also harbor the so-called mutated alleles that produce a non-functional enzyme that may then lead to albinism; I ignore for now the fact that there are also other kinds of albinism. Then there are genes that require additional steps to take effect to cause differences between people. The gene for the ABO blood type can hold an allele for antigen A or one for antigen B; these alleles produce an enzyme that then creates the corresponding A-antigens and B-antigens—which is a two-step process. Then there are genes that require many more steps, or they require the cooperation of many more genes, in order to produce different end results.

As a matter of fact, the vast majority of human diseases and other genetic traits are multi-factorial. They are influenced by a multitude of genes that interact with one another, as well as by a vast assortment of signals from the environment of each cell—such as signals from the nutrient supply, hormones, and electrical signals from other cells. All of these, together with influences that represent the external world of the organism as a whole—factors such as upbringing, learning, experience, culture, and religion—affect diseases and genetic traits. Thus the same mutation in a specific gene can actually produce very different results depending on its environment as well as the genetic background of all other interacting genes together. Each human being has a background that is unique; even identical twins, although they carry identical alleles, may turn out very differently. I would say that simplicity has turned into complexity!

How then do genes work? Since the discovery of DNA, we have a better understanding of exactly how genes operate. For a while, geneticists held on to what they literally called their "central dogma." That dogma said, "DNA makes RNA makes protein"[3]—a one-directional causal flow, with one item of code, a gene, ultimately making one item of substance, an enzyme or some other kind of

---

[3] Francis Crick, "Central dogma of molecular biology," *Nature*, 227 (1970): 561–563. In particular, he stated that genetic "information cannot be transferred back from protein to either protein or nucleic acid."

protein. Then all these proteins together made a body. However, this clockwork view has dramatically changed.[4]

Leaving aside the many obviously unknown changes to come, what is the consequence of these recent changes? First of all, the key to complexity is no longer more and more genes, but more combinations and interactions generated by fewer units of genetic code. So organisms must be explained as entire organisms, and not as a summation of genes.

Second, DNA can never do anything on its own. It is not even capable, as many still believe, of replicating itself into copies for new generations, since it is manufactured out of small molecular bits and pieces by elaborate cell machinery that includes proteins. If DNA is put in the presence of all the pieces that will be assembled into new DNA, nothing happens without the protein machinery. What in fact does happen is that the already-present DNA is copied by the surrounding cellular machinery so that new DNA strands are replicas of the old ones.[5] The process is analogous to the production of copies of a document by an office copying machine, a process that can never be described as "self-replication."

Third, DNA does not, in fact, make anything, not even enzymes and other proteins. New proteins are made by a mechanism that is itself made up of proteins. The role of DNA is to specify how amino acids are to be strung together into proteins by this synthetic machinery. But this string of amino acids is not yet a protein. To become a protein with physiological and structural functions, it must be folded into a three-dimensional configuration that is only partly based on its amino acid sequence, but is also determined by the cellular environment and by special processing proteins. Insulin for diabetics is a case in point. Recently the DNA coding sequence for human insulin has been inserted into bacteria so that they produce a protein with the amino acid sequence of human insulin. But it turned

---

[4] See Intermission 2A at the end of this chapter.

[5] DNA is a double-stranded string of nucleotides (containing A, C, T, or G). You can picture the DNA helix as a twisting ladder with rungs made of one of these four base pairs: A-T, T-A, C-G, or G-C. If you split all the pairs in half, thus cutting the ladder down the center of each rung, each half-ladder contains all the genetic information needed to rebuild a complete copy of the original—for base A will couple only with base T, and so on.

out that amino acid sequence does not determine the shape of a protein. The first proteins harvested through this process did have the correct sequence, but were physiologically inactive. Imagine! The bacterial cell had folded the protein incorrectly. That is enough to take DNA off its pedestal.

So what has happened to the belief that DNA holds the secret of life? I call such a belief the DNA mantra—a new version of determinism, this time called genetic determinism. Adherents of this view should know better; it is not that they are ignorant but that they know so much that isn't so. What then isn't so? As we found out, this "miraculous" DNA is quite powerless: It cannot replicate itself or even create a protein on its own. It needs all the help it can get from "outside." Think of viruses, which are essentially pure DNA or RNA; their DNA or RNA cannot do anything until they penetrate, like a Trojan horse, the interior of a "living" cell. Instead of saying that DNA is the secret of life, we could as well state the opposite: the surrounding life is the secret of DNA.[6] Without its surroundings, DNA couldn't do anything!

We may have initially thought that the program for living beings is located in the genes, and then in the proteins encoded by genes and their DNA. But then we found out that this DNA is "controlled" by a whole network of proteins and other cellular components, and this cellular network in turn is part of an even larger network of surrounding cells, and this larger network, the organism, is surrounded by the external world. So we also need to know the "rules" of networks that control the DNA itself. Therefore, I would say, forget the term "DNA program." DNA is more like an archive with a set of instructions, but what to use from this archive, when, how, and where, is not determined by DNA. That would be a big blow to the clockwork concept of DNA. DNA is not the clockwork mechanism that makes us "tick." Why not?

Well, claiming that we are nothing but DNA—because DNA is supposed to be all there is to life—brings us lots of troubles. Let me mention at least four pertinent philosophical problems:

1. How could DNA create itself?

---

[6] B. Commoner, "Roles of Deoxyribonucleic Acid in Inheritance," *Nature*, 202 (1964): 960-968.

2. How could DNA replicate itself?

3. How could DNA discover itself?

4. How could DNA validate itself?

Let us tackle these questions one by one.

Problem number one: if we were nothing but DNA, DNA would have to *create* itself. Just think about that issue for a moment; it would be like the miracle of a hand drawing itself; a hand may draw a picture of a hand, of course, but a hand that draws a hand cannot produce the very hand that does the drawing! The very hand that does the drawing is "more" than the hand that is being drawn on paper. Claiming differently would be a case of philosophical magic, for a cause cannot be self-caused. A cause can never cause itself, as it would have to exist before it came into existence. It certainly would be nice if gold could create itself from nothing! But we all know that is impossible. As the saying goes, "Nothing comes from nothing."

Problem number two: if we were nothing but DNA, then DNA would have to *replicate* itself. A copier makes copies, but it can never make copies of itself. Stated clearly, copying done by a copy machine is certainly not self-replication. Or take the case of a projector: it can project pictures, but it cannot project itself; self-projection is beyond the capabilities of a projector. We would need something "more" to achieve this.

Problem number three: if we were nothing but DNA, then DNA would ultimately be able to *discover* itself. If we were nothing but DNA, and some of us discovered DNA, then DNA must have discovered itself—which is certainly sheer magic again. When Watson and Crick discovered DNA, they must have been "more" than the DNA they discovered; it was certainly not their DNA that discovered DNA. This is simply logical when you think about it. How could a mirror ever mirror itself, or how could a missile ever target itself, or how could a finger ever point at itself, or how could a camera ever make pictures of itself? In order to do any of these things, we need something that "transcends" any of these items, something that is capable of doing something "more" than the item itself can achieve.

Problem number four: If we were nothing but DNA, then DNA would have to *validate* itself. Claims can be true or false, but molecules such as DNA cannot be true or false; molecules can be small or large, stable or unstable, but never true or false. In order to make any claims whatever, we need to validate our claims as being true, otherwise they are worth nothing. If we were nothing but DNA, this very statement that we are making here would not be worth more than its molecular origin, and neither would we, who are making this statement, be more than that molecular origin. Such claims just defeat and destruct themselves. They cut off the very branch that the person who makes such claims was sitting on. I consider that to be suicide!

The four problems mentioned above lead us to an important conclusion: the knowing subject, you and me, must be "more" than the known object, DNA or whatever—in the same way as a projector must be more than the pictures it projects. Perhaps I should state it even more strongly, but possibly more controversially: the physical world can never be *studied* by something purely physical!

Even Charles Darwin had some awareness of this disconcerting problem—good for him I would say!—but unfortunately he never thought it through.[7] Here is what he said in his *Autobiography*:

> [If the theory of natural selection comes from the human mind,] one might wonder whether the mind of man, which has, as I fully believe, been developed from a mind as low as that possessed by the lowest animal, [can] be trusted when it draws such grand conclusions.[8]

And again in a letter to William Graham in July 1881 he raises the question:

> ...whether the convictions of a man's mind...are of any value or at all trustworthy. Would anyone trust in the

---

[7] Curiously enough, Charles Darwin applied this to one's belief in *God* (theism) but not to his own belief in *evolution* (evolutionism). His conclusion was that we cannot trust anything we know about God, whereas I would argue the opposite — that we cannot trust anything we know at all if there were no God.

[8] Charles Darwin, *The Autobiography of Charles Darwin* (Cambridge, U.K.: Icon Books, Ltd., 2003), 149.
Or from Charles Darwin, *Autobiography*, in *The Life and Letters of Charles Darwin*, ed. Francis Darwin, vol. 1 (London: John Murray, 1888), 307.

convictions of a monkey's mind, if there are any convictions in such a mind?[9]

I certainly would not!

Think about this problem for a moment: if natural selection were the origin of all there is in life, including the human mind, it would act as a boomerang that comes back to its maker, in a vicious circle, knocking out the truth claims of whoever launched it. How could we ever trust the outcome of mere natural selection when it comes to matters of truth? In fact, the theory of natural selection must *assume* the human mind, but it can neither create it nor explain it. On its own, natural selection would be just a powerless and useless concept, for if one can't trust the rationality of human beings, one is logically prevented from having confidence in one's own rational activities—with science being one of them. Obviously, the all-inclusive claim of evolutionism has run into serious trouble in much the same way that the all-inclusive claim of determinism has. They both defeat themselves—if they are true, they become false. The trouble of such a claim is that it cuts off its very reason for reasoning and for trusting its own rationality! It would become its own undertaker. That is certainly a very haunting implication.

So in response to the question "What makes you tick?" the answer would not and could not be DNA or natural selection in and of themselves. I do admit that DNA has an impact on what you and I came to be, but it can only be part of a larger picture. I have no problem with the fact that DNA may have some determining power in life, but the fact that DNA is important doesn't necessarily make it decisive. There are in fact many genetic predispositions that we can do something about. My genetic tendency to nearsightedness is canceled by the eyeglasses I wear. Many other genetic diseases can be prevented by the use of diets or medication. With proper genetic knowledge, we can take charge of our genes so that we are no longer their victim, but rather their architect. What I do oppose is the idea that we are supposed to be completely at the mercy of DNA, making us mere victims of our genes. According to this DNA ideology, even those kinds of behavior that we think are our own choosing—lifestyle choices, moral decisions, and the like—would require us to postulate a

[9] In a letter to William Graham, author of *Creed of Science: Religious, moral, and social* (London: Keegan Paul & Co., 1881).

gene for what we do. That would amount to real "puppet determinism." Those who seriously claim this must also carry a gene that makes them think so!

In short, there must be something more than DNA that makes us "tick." Even Darwin vaguely surmised that the mind of the person who discovered the theory of evolution or the structure of DNA must be more than what was discovered. I do not think it is wise to put all our eggs in the DNA basket of evolution.

Intermission 2A

From Genes to DNA

Human beings carry 23 pairs of chromosomes—of which one pair is an "unmatched" pair in males (XY) and a "matched" pair of sex chromosomes (XX) in females. All genes are located inside these chromosomes, so they come in pairs as well. During conception, the father and the mother each contribute only half of their chromosomes, one of each pair, so their child ends up again with 23 pairs. Depending on whether the father passed on his X-chromosome or his Y-chromosome, the child will be male (XY) or female (XX). These chromosomes hold all our genes.

A decade ago, the general estimate for the number of human genes was thought to be well over 100,000, but the number turned out to be about 30,000 genes—that is only half again as many genes as a tiny roundworm needs to manufacture its utter simplicity. And we have only 300 unique genes not found in mice. No wonder that the president of a bio-corporation said about this surprising finding "This tells me genes can't possibly explain all of what makes us what we are."[1] Or as Francis Collins, the leader of the U.S. contingent to the Human Genome Project, put it:

> One surprise is just how little of the genome is actually used to code for protein.... Though limitations...prevent a precise estimate.... The total amount of DNA used by those genes to code for protein adds up to a measly 1.5 percent of the total.... Our complexity must arise not from the number of separate instruction packets, but from the way they are utilized.[2]

---

[1] Craig Venter, president of Celera Genomics, in *The San Francisco Chronicle*, February 13, 2001.

[2] Francis S. Collins, *The Language of God: A Scientist Presents Evidence for Belief* (New York: Free Press, 2006),124-125.

Due to the discovery of DNA in 1953, we have a better understanding of how exactly genes operate. As noted earlier, geneticists held on to what they called their "central dogma" that says: DNA makes RNA makes protein. But that was quite some time ago, and in the meantime we have learned that the working of DNA is much more complicated and intricate than was previously thought.

First, some DNA sections, the so-called introns, get initially transcribed into mitochondrial RNA (mRNA) but are then removed from the end product by splicing. Due to alternative splicing, a single gene may code for several different proteins. That would partially explain why the number of genes can be much lower than we initially expected.

It also turned out that protein-coding regions of genes can be interrupted by DNA segments that play more of a regulatory role by producing activator and repressor proteins that either activate or repress the activity of "regular" genes. Some of these regulatory genes are actually very short and do not produce proteins at all, but short strands of mRNA capable of blocking the mRNA of a "regular" gene from creating its protein; they are called micro-RNA-genes.

And then there was a third important discovery. Genes may be separated by long stretches of DNA that do not appear to be doing much—that is why they are often called "junk DNA," but "non-coding," "neutral," or "silent" DNA would be safer terms. Some of this "non-coding" DNA is repetitive DNA, often replicated from regular, coding DNA, and perhaps a rich source from which potentially useful new genes can emerge in evolution. An example of this would be the long cascade of blood-clotting proteins that human beings carry. Most of these have a very similar DNA structure, so it could very well be that some of them stemmed from "silent" replicated DNA sections and were then mutated. This is even more likely when we realize that fish have a much shorter cascade of blood-clotting proteins; the longer cascade of mammals has some extra proteins very similar to the original ones, but most likely a result of replicated DNA sections.

Speaking of simple genetic inheritance, the story is becoming increasingly complicated. DNA contains the genetic information that regulates the synthesis of proteins. Protein synthesis takes place in cells and typically goes through the following steps:

1. DNA in the cell nucleus acts as a template for synthesis of mRNA.

2. mRNA leaves the nucleus and enters the cytoplasm, where it complexes with ribosomes.

3. tRNA carries one specific amino acid at a time to mRNA.

4. tRNA couples briefly with mRNA on a ribosome.

5. The ribosome moves along on mRNA, adding amino acids to the growing polypeptide chain resulting in a protein.

6. tRNA moves off to pick up more amino acids.

All the steps outlined above present a very simplified version of the full story. Some DNA sections, the so-called introns, get initially transcribed into mRNA but are then removed from the end product by splicing. Introns may also contain "old code" that has become inactive. New discoveries are being made on an almost daily basis, constantly revolutionizing our current understanding of genetics.

Since just about all organisms contain DNA, comparing the DNA structure of different species may be an indication of how closely the organisms are related. The technique for making the comparisons uses DNA from two different species, and their strands are uncoupled. Next, the single-stranded DNA from the two organisms is mixed under conditions that allow them to recouple. The amount of coupling gives us a measure of the degree of genetic similarity between the two species. Indeed, DNA is like a logbook reaching almost as far back as the origin of life.

But there is even better evidence of genetic similarity than the degree of coupling; it is based on the so-called pseudo-genes. These are genes that resemble a regular DNA packet of a functional gene, but they have been affected by one or more "glitches" that change their script into "nonsense." They were once functional copies of genes, but have since lost their protein-coding ability and, presumably, their biological function as well. In a way, pseudo-genes are like rudimentary organs. When comparing humans and chimpanzees, we find genes that are functional in one species but not in the other, so we call them pseudo-genes. A striking example is the gene for a jaw-muscle protein called MYH16. This has become a pseudo-gene in humans, but is still very functional in developing strong jaw muscles in other primates. Another example would be the

DNA sequence for an enzyme that produces ascorbic acid (vitamin C) in most animals. Many primates, including humans, have a defect in this DNA code, creating the need to acquire vitamin C through food; but they did hold on to its repetitive sequences in the "silent" section of their DNA. Amazing, isn't it! Phenomena like these are difficult to explain unless we assume some kind of evolution.

Another marvelous feature of DNA research is that it lets us trace back what the DNA of our first human ancestors must have looked like. This is done by comparing the "neutral" DNA sections of two types of DNA: mitochondrial DNA and Y-chromosomal DNA. Mitochondrial DNA is passed unmixed from a mother to all her children, along the maternal line, whereas Y-chromosomal DNA is passed unmixed from a father to all his sons, along the paternal line. All lineages are identified by one or more of the so-called DNA markers that are rare mutations in non-coding DNA segments. DNA markers create a "DNA signature" or haplotype of their ancestry. These lineages are like "ancestral clans" and form haplo-groups with some specific rare mutations and then split into subgroups that have some additional markers based on other rare mutations. This kind of analysis allows us to construct a DNA family tree that has at its origin a "mitochondrial Eve" and a "Y-chromosomal Adam" representing our most recent common ancestors that have DNA markers like ours. Such a reconstruction has told us that these ancestors were living somewhere in Africa—findings that are consistent with paleontology.

Chapter 3

A Network of Neurons

If it is not just DNA that makes us tick then there must be something else that does. We learned in the previous chapter that the discoverers of DNA must be more than DNA, since the subject who does the investigation must be more than the object that is being investigated—in other words, the knowing subject must be more than the known object. What might this "more" be?

Many would say that is probably the point where the brain enters into the picture. Some call this the *mind*, but I would point out that what they usually mean is the brain. Neuroscience is more often than not understood as brain-science. Neuroscience has taught us more and more about this ingenious and intricate brain instrument that makes you and me number one in the animal world as far as intelligence is concerned. Well, here we have our new mantra: "brain power" has got to be the mechanism that really makes us tick!

Of course, the brain is partly determined by our DNA, but at the same time it is many steps away from DNA in the sense that there are many interfering factors that make the brain what it is. Because the end result, the phenotype, is many steps away from the genotype, the DNA, it allows for many inroads from the environment. It is due to this interaction of multiple factors—genetic as well as environmental ones—that we develop brains different from one another. And this process keeps going on and on. The brain affects our behavior, but this behavior, in turn, again affects the brain. A similar phenomenon is well known from sports, for instance: strong muscles benefit those who play sports, but in turn, playing sports greatly benefits the development of muscles. In regard to environmental reinforcing conditions, consider that being an only child or being the first child can make a huge difference in growing up.

The outcome of this growth process is that we each have our very own unique brain makeup. Even identical twins have gone through their own individual growth process, so they may differ dramatically in phenotype, in spite of the fact that they do have the same genotype. And even if they are act-alikes or look-alikes, that could very well be the result of their *desire* to be alike. No wonder the brain is considered an important part of what makes us tick. In the words of the DNA co-discoverer Francis Crick, "You're nothing but a pack of neurons."[1] That is the latest offshoot of determinism.

What does this "network of neurons" look like? Scientists often speak in terms of a neuronal network—a fancy set of cogwheels. We can even compare this network with what is going on in a computer. These days, the computer has replaced the clock and watch as the latest contraption that makes us tick. To be sure, such a comparison seems attractive, since the brain does work in the same way as a computer operates, as both use a binary code based on "ones" (1) and "zeros" (0); neurons either do (1) or do not (0) fire an electric impulse—in the same way as transistors either do (1) or do not (0) conduct an electric current. So it looks as if the brain "thinks" like a computer "thinks"; and it must be this very stream of binary code in a neuronal network that makes us tick?

We should question, though, whether the above view is really true. Whatever is happening in the brain—say, some particular thought—may have a material substrate that works as a binary code, but it would not really matter whether this material substrate works with impulses as in the brain, or with currents as in a computer. Because this material is only its physical carrier, a vehicle that carries something else in the way trains transport people or goods. One and the same thought could be coded in Morse code, Braille, hieroglyphics, or any code language—even impulses. It doesn't really matter what kind of code, since these codes are just physical carriers or vehicles.

However, once we acknowledge that the same thought can be transported by different vehicles—such as pen strokes, sound waves, cogwheels, currents, impulses—we immediately realize that a thought must be different from its carrier. If I were to break my radio, the news report will stop, but this doesn't mean the news was created by the radio; it was only the vehicle that broke down. So it seems to me that the brain carrier doesn't create thoughts but merely transports

---

[1] See Francis Crick, *The Astonishing Hypothesis* (New York: Charles Scribner's Sons, 1994).

them. The thoughts somehow "use" the vehicle. The mind somehow "uses" the brain.

So what is it that sets the thought apart from its carrier? Well, thoughts are more than a binary code; they also have sense and meaning, syntax and semantics, and that is what the binary code really carries. We do not just think; we must always think *something*. Thoughts are about something else, something mental, which is something beyond themselves.

As noted by John Searle it is this very "aboutness" that a computer lacks; anything that shows up on a computer monitor remains just an "empty" collection of "ones and zeros" that do not point beyond themselves until some kind of human interpretation gives sense and meaning to the code and interprets it as being about something else.[2] Think of a picture: a picture may carry information, but the picture itself is just a piece of paper that makes "sense" only when human beings interpret the picture. The same with books: they provide lots of information for "bookworms," but to real worms they have only paper to offer. Even a banknote would just be a blank note, a worthless piece of paper, if humans didn't have a mental conception of money.

Therefore we should not idolize computers as equivalents of human brains. When Marvin Minsky, a pioneer in the field of artificial intelligence but certainly not in philosophy, refers to human beings as mere meat-machines or machines made of meat, he had just "forgotten" that computers require a human maker and would still need a human subject to give their informational output some meaning or sense. Without human subjects, computers cannot "think." Computers do not create thoughts, but they may carry thoughts that were created by the mind of a human subject—for example, when using a word-processing program. Consider a voice

---

[2] The term "aboutness" has become common parlance through the writings of John Searle, who argues that intentionality is the "aboutness" of the mind to things, objects, states of affairs, events—even if these do not exist in the outside world. He used this concept also in his "Chinese Room Argument" against the feasibility of artificial intelligence. See his *Intentionality: An Essay on the Philosophy of Mind* (Cambridge: Cambridge University Press, 1983) and his *The Rediscovery of Mind* (Cambridge, MA: The MIT Press, 1992).

recognition system; it doesn't really understand what it is programmed to "recognize." Computers do only what we, human beings with a mind, cause them do, for we have proven to be champion machine builders. A computer may play chess better than Garry Kasparov or any other champion, but it plays the game for the same "reason" a calculator adds or a pump pumps—the reason being that it is a machine designed for that purpose and not because it "wants" to or is "happy" to do so. Why not? Well, a machine doesn't have an "I" behind it—other than the "I" of its maker. No matter what I think when I am thinking, it is always "I" who is thinking something.

With regard to the man-machine interface, some may have settled for the idea that man is just a machine, but a better concept is something like "a man using the machine." For without human input, machines are merely meaningless tools. Without a human subject, objects do not have any meaning, do not make any sense, and do not even exist—for these objects are objects of knowledge, that is, mental concepts in the human mind. The computer is the modern equivalent of clocks and watches, but it is based on the same kind of imagery, this time borrowed from the latest technology. It is a technological piece that feeds our imagery but certainly limits our imagination.

We should also clarify the relationship of the mind to "network of neurons," the mind-brain interface. For, as we discovered earlier, the knowing subject must be more than the known object. So how should we consider the brain? It is the *known* object! And what then is the *knowing* subject? Not the brain but the mind! Without a human mind as a subject, there wouldn't be any mental objects at all—not even the object that we create in our minds of what we call a neuronal network. Computers, radios, and other devices do not have meaning or sense in themselves until a human subject uses them as carriers of information that receives sense and meaning from a human subject. For those who like images and analogies: the mind uses the brain in the way a programmer would use a computer.

Isn't this dualism, you might ask? No, all that is being stressed is that the "knowing subject" is "more than" any "known object." All knowledge of objects is based on a subject that apprehends those objects, *but the subject itself can never be fully captured by making it an object.* The body belongs to the world of objects, whereas the mind is part of the world of subjects. The body has characteristics such as length, width, height, and weight, but the mind doesn't have any of those; thoughts are true or false, right or wrong, but they are never tall or short, heavy or light. Therefore body and mind are two different aspects of the same human being; you can tell them apart but you can't *set* them apart.

Once we realize this, we have to change the way we think and talk about the human brain and the human mind. One would need a mind before one can study the brain! Unfortunately, we have been 'brainwashed' to think that the mind is nothing but the brain. However, when studying the human brain, neuroscientists make the human brain an object of science, but they can only do so because they have a human mind that is the subject behind science. Without the human mind, there would be no science. Sure, the human mind uses the human brain, but it is also more than the human brain.

Let us analyze the difference between mind and body a bit further by quoting an observation that was made by the famous philosopher Ludwig Wittgenstein.[3] Picture yourself watching through a mirror how a scientist is studying your opened skull for "brain waves." Wittgenstein once noted correctly that the scientist is observing just one thing—outer brain activities—but the "brain-owner" is actually observing two things—the outer brain activities via the mirror as well as the inner thought processes that no one else has access to. In order for them to make the connection between "inner" mental states and "outer" neural states, scientists would depend on information that only the "brain-owner" can provide. And if you argue that the same theory holds true for pain, I would point out that pain can be induced physically, whereas thoughts cannot.

Imagine that someone purported to give you a full scientific description of the status of your mind at this moment after making a scan of your brain. No matter what, this description would ultimately depend on whether you believe it or not, because the simple act of your acceptance or rejection would change your brain's makeup—and no scan can predict this act.[4] The search for a complete description of my brain's makeup defeats itself, because complete knowledge would

---

[3] Ludwig Wittgenstein, *The Blue And Brown Book* (New York: Harper & Row, 1980).

[4] More on this in Donald MacKay, *Science and the Quest for Meaning* (Grand Rapids, Mich: Eerdmans, 1982), 21-25.

not only entail full knowledge of all surrounding factors involved but also full knowledge of my knowledge itself, and the knowledge of this knowledge, and so on and on—which would lead to infinite regress. So do not equate a description of your brain with a description of your mind. The mind that creates thoughts must be more than the thoughts it creates.

Let us explore what infinite regress means. A series of propositions leads to infinite regress if the truth of the first one requires the support of a second one, the truth of the second one requires the support of a third one, and so on, and the truth of the next-to-last one requires the support of the last one, where the number of "last" approaches infinity. What is wrong with infinity? Infinity sounds counter-intuitive, but with infinities routinely manipulated in mathematics, it is difficult to reject an infinity as such. So some cases of infinite regress may not be "vicious," but others are—although the distinction is often hard to make. A vicious regress is an attempt to solve a problem by re-introducing the same problem in the proposed solution, which makes for a circular argument that begs the question. It explains a phenomenon in terms of the very phenomenon it is supposed to explain. If one continues along the same lines, the initial problem will recur infinitely and will never be solved. Take the following reference in a dictionary: "Circle: See 'Circle.' " Every step toward a goal somehow leaves the goal removed by another step. Somehow, some supposed end remains unattained. Something similar happens when we try to give a complete description of someone's brain makeup.

Let us go back to our distinction between mind and brain. This distinction has quite some implications. Do not confuse a "defective brain" with a "broken mind." Even people who have "lost their mind," so to speak (through dementia, Alzheimer's disease, autism, or insanity), haven't really lost their minds or their souls, but they have lost parts of their brains; there happen to be certain defects in the physical network of neurons or neurotransmitters that prevent the mind from working through bodily activities the way it used to, or usually does. It compares to the static noise in a news broadcast. In that sense, Stephen Hawking, the theoretical physicist and cosmologist, may be right when he regards the brain as a computer that will stop working when its components fail.[5] In such cases, the mind has become an incarcerated mind working with a failing brain. However, therapy may often help such people to stay in touch with their "self." What comes to mind are also individuals with a speech impediment, or people who are seemingly in a coma; they just cannot say what they want to say. "Mind over matter" may not work at all times, since "matter" sometimes just won't "cooperate" with the mind. Recall our comparison with a radio? The radio doesn't produce news reports but just carries and broadcasts them. So do not overlook what is behind the carrier.

It is true that in response to certain thoughts some brain areas may appear more active, but that doesn't necessarily mean that those areas produce the thought; all we can say is that they probably carry the thought. Simply put, thoughts are more than brain waves, in the same way that love is more than a chemical reaction. Professionals can read and interpret an electroencephalogram (EEG), but looking at it doesn't show them any thoughts.[6]

The question remains, of course, how mind and matter can interact if they are so different. Since the mind does not occur on the physical, scientific map of the body, it may seem to be nowhere in the chain of bodily activities, yet it is the "soul" of it all and pervades the entire body; it is "part" of everything the body does without being a bodily part.

The body-mind relationship is complicated and mind-boggling! Obviously, body and mind do not have a mental relationship; on the other hand, it is not a physical relationship either. Thoughts may make you cry, but certainly not in the physical way that cutting an onion makes you cry. And crying may make you think, but there is certainly not a physical causation here. Bodily activities, for their part, are undeniably connected in a physical way; a lot of running physically causes you to eat. Mental activities, on the other hand, are mentally related. Thinking of "two times zero" doesn't physically cause the thought of "zero" (plenty of nothing is still nothing); we

---

[5] Stephen Hawking, "There is no heaven; it's a fairy story" Interview with Ian Sample, science correspondent, *The Guardian* May 15, 2011.

[6] This is very different from pain and other sensations; those can be physically induced with electrodes, but such a thing is not possible for thoughts, since they are of a different nature.

may wish it did, so we could have skipped many years of schooling and education. Thinking of "E" doesn't physically make us think of "mc²." The thought of "malaria" doesn't physically evoke the thought of "mosquitoes"; that link comes from research. The thought of "smoking tobacco" and the thought of "lung cancer" are not physically connected; making such a connection requires awareness and some education.

Therefore, we should never degrade the mind's activity to a physical link in a network of physical causes among neurons, muscles, and so on. Blinking an eye is usually a reflex, a process based on physical causes, but *winking* at someone is certainly different from blinking an eye, as it adds an intention to the process and surpasses a series of physical causes. We are able to control the physical causes behind blinking by having the intention of winking, but it eludes us how the mind and its intentions interact with the brain. It is, of course, notable that if thoughts were really the product of bodily actions, all thoughts would be equivalent to one another, and we would have no way of telling true from false, or knowledge from error. Apparently the mind is not one of the players on the neuronal scene, but instead it is the author as well as the producer behind this neuronal play. The mind can create its own non-physical causes in the midst of physical causes.

As mentioned earlier, the mind does interfere with physical causes, but it does so in a rather mysterious way: The mental and physical aspects affect each other in a way similar to the mysterious way mass and gravity affect each other; we just do not know the "mechanism" of their interaction, and yet their interaction is somehow part of the cosmic design of creation. We just lack understanding of what it is that enables our minds to understand this world through what happens in the brain. But no matter what or how, humans definitely are "self-moved movers," altering themselves and their surroundings through decisions they make, and through values they hold in their mysterious minds. Thoughts can and do move the world, as we all know; they make us "tick." But how can this possibly happen?

Let us clarify this issue by using an example from sports. When golfers hit the ball, or when baseball hitters make contact with the pitcher's ball, they apply the laws of physics—that is, they apply a specific force at a certain angle that has a specific impact, and so on.

We have a cascade of physical causes and effects here. And yet there is much more going on in this process—these players have a very specific intention in mind, which eludes and transcends the laws of science. Do they go against the laws of nature? Of course they do not; but they do go *beyond* those laws. People who can't look beyond those physical laws and causes are completely missing out on what the game is about.

Apparently we are entering here a metaphysical territory located beyond the physical domain.[7] Since the mind is not one of the players on the neuronal scene, but instead is the author as well as the producer behind this neuronal play, we are back again at that famous question Charles Darwin posed long ago, but never answered. Darwin's question was: Can science as carried out by a human brain be trusted if that science is found to be the outcome of some evolutionary process of natural selection? Now we know what the answer must look like: science was developed by the human mind, but the human mind is more than the human brain; a mental state of the mind is more than a neural state of the brain. The brain may be a product of natural selection, but that doesn't mean the mind is too. It is worth quoting again and noting exactly how Darwin worded, and thus obscured, his problem:

> One might wonder whether the *mind* of man, which has, as I fully believe, been developed from a *mind* as low as that possessed by the lowest animal, [can] be trusted when it draws such grand conclusions (emphasis added).[8]

In both cases, he should have used the word *brain* instead of *mind*. The brain may have developed from the animal kingdom, but the mind is

---

[7] Metaphysics is a branch of philosophy concerned with explaining the fundamental nature of being and the world. The term was first used as the title for several of Aristotle's works, because they were usually placed after the works on physics in complete editions. The prefix *meta*—("beyond") indicates that these works come "after" the chapters on physics. However, Aristotle did not call the subject of these books "Metaphysics," but referred to it as "First Philosophy."

[8] Charles Darwin, *The Autobiography of Charles Darwin* (Cambridge, U.K.: Icon Books, Ltd., 2003), 149.
Or from Charles Darwin, *Autobiography* (1876), in *The Life and Letters of Charles Darwin*, ed. Francis Darwin, vol. 1 (London: John Murray, 1888), 307.

not a product of evolution. If it were, we definitely should be questioning the validity of our knowledge—which necessarily includes our scientific knowledge of the very theory of evolution.

Let us come to a conclusion. Without the mind, we couldn't study the brain. It is the mind that makes us tick, not just the brain. So we need to find out what the mind is if it is supposed to be more than the brain. Beyond physical realm of space and time science has no answers to questions that arise. This journey will take us beyond the realm of physics into the domain of metaphysics.

Intermission 3A

What Makes Mental Concepts Unique

Human beings have a mental concept of what a physical thing is and what it can do; it is through mental concepts that they can transform "things" of the world into "objects" of knowledge. This is not so with animals. If we train a dog to associate a command like "The boss!" with its real boss, then that dog has been conditioned to respond to the command "The boss!" by looking for the real boss. The sound "Boss" has become a *signal* for the "real thing." Signals depend on the actual presence of the "real thing." The dog has a physical image of its boss, but it has no mental concept of what *a boss* is like. Human beings certainly share this feature with animals; one employee yelling "The boss!" is actually signaling all others present to start looking extremely busy. That is what signals do. Monkeys, for instance, have different signals for different types of enemies, but they use them only when such an enemy is around; they do not just "ponder" and "chat" about their enemies.

But what is unique in humans is the fact that they can also use the phrase "the boss" as a *symbol* for a "mental object" of a boss; in fact, when they use that phrase, the real boss may not be around, or they may only do so when the real boss is in fact physically absent. Instead, they use their "mental object" of a boss to debate, for example, why their real boss doesn't qualify as a boss, or which real boss they would prefer instead. In other words, they are actually comparing the "real thing" (perhaps far away) with a "mental object." Mental concepts transform "things" of the world into "objects" of knowledge, thus enabling humans to see with their "mental eyes" what no physical eyes could ever see before. While animals live in a world of events, humans also inhabit a world of facts—which are mental interpretations of those events. Events may be the "physical" parts of our world, but facts are "mental" creations—the interpretations of events in our minds. There are no facts without interpretation.

41

Let us take an example of what this entails as far as facts are concerned. The more interpretation we inject into facts, the more information we can provide, but we also increase what requires to be proven. When I describe a certain event taking place in the sky by saying "those are moving spots," I express relatively "empty" information, but it is rather "safe" information. When I say, however, "Those are flying birds," I convey more information—and therefore I may need to come up with more evidence to support my claim. And when I say, "Those are migrating geese," I inflate my information even more, thus making my factual statement still more vulnerable to falsification. So what is the "real" fact here, one may ask—is it moving spots or flying birds or migrating geese, or perhaps none of these? Only further investigation can tell us what the right interpretation of the event is.

In short, without concepts there wouldn't be any facts, for facts are the objects of our thoughts. Imagine where science would be without facts and the use of hypotheses! The answer is "nowhere," for these are based on mental concepts.

Intermission 3B

Are We the Only Rational Beings on Earth?

When it comes to intelligence, we do not seem to be exceptional creatures. I realize that intelligence is a rather complex entity; it has many faces—social, practical, formal, spatial, and so on. Yet, all animals show some form of intelligence in their behavior, because intelligence is a brain feature and as such it is an important tool in survival. That is why animals show various forms of intelligence. To name just a few, we find spatial intelligence in pigeons and bats, social intelligence in wolves and monkeys, formal intelligence in apes and dolphins, and practical intelligence in rats and ravens.

But let us not go overboard! Almost a century ago Edward Thorndike the pioneer of American experimental psychology complained bitterly in 1911 about the books of his day that were published after Darwin. He said they gave:

> ...not a psychology, but rather a eulogy of animals. They have all been about animal intelligence, never about animal stupidity.[1]

He was right; there's certainly a lot of "stupidity" in the animal world when it comes to formal intelligence.

Just think of the following cases:

- The cat that was placed in a closed box, and then discovered after many trials how to pull a cord in order to open an escape hole, still keeps pulling the cord before crawling out, even when the escape hole is already open.

- The cat that had finally learned to escape by pulling a cord, but when subsequently placed in the same box without the

---

[1] Edward L. Thorndike, *Animal Intelligence* (New York: Macmillan Co., 1911), 22.

cord, goes through the motions of pawing the air where the cord had been before.

- The elephants that had learned to lift a lid to retrieve food from a bucket didn't "get it" when the lid was placed alongside the bucket while the food was simultaneously placed inside the bucket; all trained elephants continued to toss the lid before retrieving the reward, raising the possibility that they have no understanding of this simple causal relationship.

- The chimpanzee that doesn't know how to remove an obstacle in order to reach food.

- The chimpanzee that has learned to invoke help from a trainer but does not know which trainer to call upon if one of them has a bucket over his head while the other has not.

- And my favorite one, the chimpanzee that cannot learn to secure a larger reward by pointing to a smaller one. The immediate urge for food just overrules any intelligent alternatives.

So animals may have different degrees of intelligence, but certainly not of the high standard found in humans. Why is it that animal intelligence so often disappoints us? Could it be the fact that animals lack rationality, in addition to intelligence? Rationality is different from intelligence; intelligence may provide some helpful survival tools, but ultimately it is our rationality that allows us to understand and explain the world we live in by the use of mental concepts.

Yet there are scientists who assert that animals must have some rationality. According to their ideas, the difference between animals and humans has got to be one of degree, not of kind. Obviously, it remains a perpetual temptation to interpret animal behavior in terms of rationality—which is done by equating motives and instincts to reasons, where instincts are the innate, inherent inclinations of a living organism toward a particular behavior. Animals often do have motives and instincts, for instance the drive to migrate, or just to cross a river. But this doesn't necessarily imply that they make reasoned decisions as well. Animals can even react to the drives of other animals, but that doesn't mean they can "read each other's minds." All this can be explained by saying that they learned to associate certain behaviors with certain outcomes—but we must not confuse this with rationality.

Something similar holds for those animals that, depending on their intelligence, show some capability of seeing "physical" connections between things. Because of this, animals are able to perform trial-and-error activities. Chimpanzees, for instance, have been able to "see" that a stick can help them reach food by making such a "physical" connection when they see a stick near food; but if the food and the stick are kept far apart, they cannot make the connection—even if they were able to do so previously. Apparently the stick is not a mental concept, but rather a physical signal that can invoke an intelligent reaction; a chimpanzee may have a physical image of a stick in relationship to food, but it has no mental concept of what a stick is and what it can do in various situations.

We can describe the animal behavior more generally by noting that animals are fully enveloped in their surroundings; they are not subjects capable of creating mental objects transcending the immediate situation. Animals are caught up in a network of physical connections, unable to transcend the current situation with the mental power of abstract concepts and reasoning. This explains a fundamental difference between intelligence and rationality.

Humans, on the other hand, can do trial-and-error operations in their mind before they give it an actual trial. For example, the human mind of a tool maker is able to create tools according to some mental concept of a tool object with which they constantly compare the real product they are working on. Thus they anticipate the future by means of abstract rational conceptions residing in their minds. The human mind is able to conceive of an object's properties and relationships in various situations, and this is exactly the point where rationality differs from intelligence. Humans are masters of "envision-ation"; they can form a picture in their minds, in their imagination, envisioning things that do not yet exist.

Let us come to a conclusion. Are we the only thinkers on planet Earth? When it comes to intelligence, humans may not be the only thinkers here on Earth; they are arguably the greatest by far. But humanity is not measured by intelligence, since intelligence is just a matter of good brain-wiring. More intelligence doesn't make us more human, but rationality does make us human. When it comes to rationality, human thinkers seem to occupy a very lonely position, because rationality is a feature of the human mind, not of a brain.

It is the human mind that has this unique ability to think under the guidance of the light of reason, taking the world as something created according to an intelligible plan accessible to the human intellect through the natural light of reason. Think of science, a rational enterprise *par excellence,* or of any philosophical system, or of any religious beliefs: all of these require intricate mental and rational concepts and therefore are not products of intelligence but of rationality.

So to answer our original question—are we the only rational beings on Earth? I would say we are not the only intelligent beings, but we certainly are the only rational beings around.

Chapter 4

Thoughts, Hopes, and Dreams

In the previous chapter, I made some controversial statements: The brain may carry your thoughts, hopes, and dreams, but it is the mind that creates them. My claim is that the neural network is the carrier for mental objects but does not produce them. Another way of saying this is as follows: it is not my brain, but it is "I", who has thoughts, reasons, goals, intentions, hopes, and dreams. All these exist only in "the I of the beholder." It is "I" who really makes me tick. So who or what is this "I"? Is it just what some have sarcastically called "a ghost in the machine"?[1]

There is something very enigmatic about this "I." You may, for instance, think "I cannot help what I do, for the activity of my brain cells is determined by physical and biological laws." However, it is your very "I" who is thinking this! Is such a thought also determined by those physical and biological laws? Somehow, we are talking here at two very different levels. In my thoughts, I am always a step "ahead" or "above" myself—which has been called the "systematic elusiveness of I," leaving science behind "in the dust." This then leads us to the question as to what this so-called systematic elusiveness of "I" is. We are leaving physical territory here and are entering the metaphysical realm.

In recent history, metaphysics has been under attack, especially from those who are in the camps of positivism, logical-positivism, and linguistic analysis. According to these opponents of metaphysics, metaphysics violates elemental rules of speaking and thinking when it tries to explain the fundamental nature of being and the world. It is their viewpoint that language should be either empirical (dealing with facts, like in science) or logical (adhering to rules, like in logic

---

[1] Gilbert Ryle [1949], *The Concept of Mind* (New University of Chicago Press edition 2002). He also coined the expression "the systematic elusiveness of I."

and mathematics), otherwise it is considered a nonsensical abuse of language; hence metaphysics amounts to uttering nonsense.

A problem with such attacks is that they determine ahead of time the outcome they like to see. They define what is legitimate by making sure they exclude what they do not want to be legitimate. Besides, I ask whether this claim in itself is either logical or empirical. We must be on guard against those who would contemptuously dismiss as meaningless those concepts whose meanings elude them! Finally, I reiterate that all claims against metaphysics are themselves essentially metaphysical viewpoints. So I would say, let us go beyond the horizon of physics, as indeed do those who deny metaphysics, into the domain of some healthy metaphysics.

When asking myself the question "Who am I?" I am certainly not doing so from a desire to find out my own name, gender, age, and so on. Instead, I am searching for something "behind" these personal details—something unique that does not and cannot belong to anyone else. And yet we cannot put our finger on what this "I" stands for. It is like my shadow—always a pace ahead of me, leaving open what the next step will be. The shadow of oneself will never wait to be jumped on; it evades capture, and yet is never very far ahead.

It is here that we come in touch with this astounding capability of the human mind—its capacity of reflecting on its "self." I may notice, for instance, that I am clumsy; I may even notice that I am laughing at myself for being clumsy; and then I may decide to tell others that I noticed how I was laughing at my own clumsiness. This is in fact an iterative or recursive process of self-reflection, making "I" act like my own shadow. I can never get away from it in the same way that I can get away from someone else's shadow. When I reflect on myself, it is always "I" doing this. Imagine a missile being its own target, or your index finger pointing at itself. Impossible, I would say! Yet it is "I" who can do so; "I" can think about myself, correct my own actions, comment on my own actions, and even revise the comments on my own actions. In short, I have this unique desire to learn about myself, about my own "self," through self-reflection.

We have a fascinating situation here: I-as-a-subject (I-now) can reflect on I-as-an-object (I-past). As a subject, I may investigate I-as-an-object and then realize, for instance, that I-as-an-object made a mistake. In contrast, I-as-a-subject is never open to investigation, because its future possibilities are beyond its current actualities—and therefore, I-now is always a pace ahead of I-past. I can remember my past only because I-now is "more" than I-past. That is why I can never blame my "glands" or my animal ancestry for what I do wrong, because I-now is always a pace ahead of I-past, including my glands. "I as an object" is my body, which may appear in the iron grip of determinism, but "I as a subject" is my mind, free to take a next step, a step ahead of any determinism.

Whenever I reflect on myself as an object, there is "some I" doing all of this as a subject. When reflecting further on this very "I," there is another "I," a new I-now, "looking over the shoulder" of I-past. Compare this with the following plain situation: a painter in a room could never make a painting of everything in that room, for such a painting should include the painter himself as well as the painting itself, which would be a painting of a painting, and on and on. This is a form of infinite regress of the vicious type.

Each time that I-now as a subject tries to catch I-past as an object, I-now stays ahead of the game, because I-as-a-subject is a necessary condition for comprehending any objects whatsoever, including I-as-an-object. Objects are based on mental conceptions residing in the human mind. Put differently, the mind is not an object like other objects in this world, but it is their very origin; without the mind, there wouldn't be any objects of knowledge comprehensible to us. I cannot help but conclude that the human mind is an elusive entity in this universe; no wonder that it is called immaterial and spiritual, in contrast to the material and physical nature of the brain.

There is another aspect of human self-reflection and self-awareness that I need to discuss: the human mind has the capacity of transcending even itself. When I say or think "I am only human," I am not comparing myself with something "below" me, such as a cat, a dog, or an ape. No, I am comparing myself with something—or rather someone—"above" me and transcending me. When I call myself "only human," I am actually comparing myself with someone who does not have the limitations I experience myself—my Maker perhaps? In some mysterious way, I am reaching out into the realm of the Absolute, far beyond myself. In so doing, the "finite" catches a glimpse of the Infinite.

Of course, I cannot transcend myself on my own, but because I myself was made in the image of Someone "above" me, I perceive more than myself whenever I perceive myself completely. Apparently

Homo sapiens is at the same time also a *Homo religiosus.* My brain may make me a genius, but my mind could turn me into a sage.

Indeed, the human mind has the amazing ability to reach beyond its own body, or even beyond the universe, stepping into the domain of the "Grand Beyond." It can only do so if the human mind is a "take-off" of its Maker's Mind. Since we were created in God's image and likeness, we have been endowed with rationality and morality, a fact that sets us apart from the rest of the living world. Here we stumble upon another elusive part of the human mind and soul. I would say it is our very humanity that is at stake here. No wonder science had to drop out of the race long ago, for even if science wants to study the human mind, it needs to start from the minds of those very scientists. So biology may some day perhaps fully understand the human brain, but it can never fully comprehend the human mind, because biology itself depends on the working of the human mind. I consider that mind-boggling.

And then there is another aspect of the human mind that I would stress. The world of the mind is a private world. Mental events happen in my private world which I have exclusively to myself, a world to which no one else has direct access. Whereas the world of my body is public and accessible to others, the world of my mind is private. It is through introspection and retrospection that I have access to my own private world in a way no one else has. Introspection and retrospection are essentially the same: I-now reflecting on I-past. This privacy aspect is, of course, intimately related to the prior discussion on elusiveness.

Even brain scans have no access to my private world like I myself do; all they can pick up are "brain waves," but never my thoughts, for those fail to show up on pictures and scans. The German philosopher Gottfried Leibniz once suggested picturing the brain so much enlarged that one could walk in it as if in a mill.[2] Inside, we would only observe movements of several parts, but never anything like a thought. For this reason, he concluded that thoughts must be different from physical and material movements and parts. How could the physical world ever be studied by something purely physical? Studying what is physical requires someone supra-physical

---

[2] Gottfried Leibniz (1646–1716), *Monadology* (Charleston, SC: Forgotten Books, 2008), section 17.

or trans-physical, which certainly takes us into the metaphysical realm.

We live in a world of what is "seen and unseen," "visible and invisible." The things that can be "seen" always occupy a certain place, they are tied to a certain time frame, they are transitory, as they will be gone some day, they are subject to change, they could have been different, or could not have existed at all; in other words, they are contingent. Hence all that is "seen" in this world is characterized by being in a certain space and a certain time frame; it comes into being, changes, and passes away, it is individual and not "necessary."

Well, it is in the middle of this comfortable, spacious, temporal, transient, and piecemeal world that laws "pop up"—physical and biological laws, mathematical laws, as well as moral laws. Laws do not have any of the above-mentioned features—none. A law is not located somewhere, not even in my mind, for that is just a mental picture of the law, but a law is everywhere. It is also beyond time, a timeless entity that can't emerge, nor can it perish. Neither are laws subject to change, for they will always remain true, even before we knew them. And here is the most important difference: not only are laws general, as we find the same law applied all over the universe, over and over again, but they are also necessary, which means that things cannot be different from what is expressed in laws.

Apparently the inhabitants of the immaterial world are very different from the inhabitants of the material world. Laws are very different from all that is "seen" around us. They belong to a different world—a "virtual" world of thoughts and truths, so to speak. Unlike the things that can be "seen," laws are not three-dimensional, temporal, transient, individual, and contingent. Don't they look like ghosts from the outer-world? Wouldn't it be much simpler if we could make them disappear, or transform them, so they become fundamentally identical to all other regular things in this physical universe? Some thinkers, such as David Hume, have certainly tried to do this by claiming that laws are just mental creations. If so, laws would exist only in the minds of mathematicians, physicists, and ethicists. However, this solution fails to explain that laws really hold in the real world. How is it possible for a bridge that has been designed according to the right laws to stand firm, while another bridge collapses because its engineer erred in his calculations? How could these laws ever hold if they were only creations of our minds?

Therefore, I would argue that laws can't easily be bypassed in that fashion. They are not material but immaterial—call them mental, spiritual, or whatever you prefer. I am reluctant to call them mental, for that adjective might suggest that they exist only in our minds. On the contrary, they are very "real" and exist outside the mind. We may know them but we do not create them; they have to be discovered, not invented. If you insist that they are created by a mind, then it is not by the human mind but by the Divine Mind—the Mind of a rational God who respects reason. Without such "given" laws, our minds would not be able to tell true from false and right from wrong. Or to quote a famous scientist, the late astrophysicist Sir James Jeans, "The universe begins to look more like a great thought than a great machine."[3] I would even dare to say that all blows aimed at our knowledge of God are blows at knowledge, at science, and at the rationality of the universe.

So in addition to a world of all that is "seen," there is an "unseen" world. Our senses give us access to all that is visible, but our thoughts give us access to what is invisible—a world of what is true in a rational sense and what is right in a moral sense. Despite this clear distinction, it remains an ongoing temptation for many scientists to reduce the mental to the neural—which amounts to what C. S. Lewis dubbed "nothing-buttery."[4] It is a claim that reduces mental states of the mind to mere neural states of the brain; it replaces the mind with the brain, the "unseen" world with the "seen" world. However, the mind doesn't go away when we try to explain it away as mere brain tissue. If the mental were the same as the neural, thoughts could never be right or wrong and true or false, because neural events simply happen, and that is that!

This takes us back again to that inescapable "systematic elusiveness of 'I'" which is inaccessible to anyone but myself. I realize that the British philosopher Gilbert Ryle sarcastically calls all this the

---

[3] James Jeans, *The Mysterious Universe* (Cambridge University Press, 1930), Chap. 5.

[4] C. S. Lewis, *The Weight of Glory and Other Addresses* (New York: Macmillan, 1980, rev. edition), 71-72.

"ghost in the machine" theory, but no matter what we call it, there is definitely something enigmatic about this situation that no one can set aside by talk or take away from us.

But there is another aspect to the human mind that needs discussing, and that is self-expression. The human mind has the astounding capacity of expressing itself in various forms of art—in literature, in painting, in music. We find these expressions as far back as the early history of humankind. Of all animals in prehistory, only humans left stones behind with inscriptions; only humans dress themselves up, and so on. And then we have the astonishing art in prehistoric caves. Understandably, evolutionists for a while considered such paintings fake because they could not accept such a high level of self-expression that early in human history. My response would be, "Even a cave man can do it!" Some of the first Cro-Magnon sites, dating from well over 30,000 years ago, have even yielded evidence for music: multi-holed bone flutes capable of producing a remarkable complexity of sound.

In addition, we see in primeval history the evidence of elaborate burials; the amount of effort put into the aesthetic productions found in prehistoric graves suggests that decoration and art were an integral part of the lives and societies of the people who made them. Besides, burial of the dead with grave goods indicates a belief in an after-life, for the goods are there because they are considered useful to the deceased in their future lives.

How far had these people come, given their assumed animal ancestry? How different this is from female apes that continue carrying their dead newborns around for quite a while, without having any idea of what is happening until finally they give up and drop the dead remains of the baby. In Guinea, West Africa, for instance, chimpanzee mothers have been observed in nature carrying and grooming their offspring's lifeless bodies for up to *sixty-eight days*. By the time the corpses were finally abandoned, the bodies had mummified and developed an intense smell of decay. Believe it or not, evolutionists give this observation a peculiar twist: these, they said, must be sixty-eight days of actually mourning the dead! All I can say in reply is that only human beings could come up with such an explanation. I would consider this sixty-eight-day period not a time of mourning, but rather a time of *ignorance*. Besides, I would ask such evolutionists where the burial and the grave are after this period of "mourning." Apparently only the "finite" human mind is able to catch a glimpse of the Infinite!

Let us not forget that only humans are able to laugh and cry, which is another sign of self-expression. Crocodiles may shed tears while devouring their prey, but we can be certain it is not because of remorse. Why are tears of laughing and crying so unique to human beings? The answer is that only humans have self-awareness and can therefore express themselves this way. If you tell me that we developed these human features only by just mimicking others, I ask you why our pets did not grab their chances then to become act and look-alikes of their owners. Are we overlooking something? Yes. The very "I of the beholder"?

There is one more striking feature of the human mind that deserves attention—its capacity for self-determination. Unlike animals, human beings have the strong desire to become someone of their own making—they *choose* their destiny. True, animals may have drives, impulses, instincts, or motives, but these are different from intentions or reasons, and they are always directly or indirectly related to sex or food. No wonder that behavioral experiments with animals usually enforce behavior with food rewards.

Humans, on the other hand, have many more kinds of goals in life; not only do they live their lives based on role models, but they also steer their lives guided by reasons, plans, convictions, beliefs, hopes, and dreams, and these shape them in how they are going to be. How different this is from animals. In the course of its life, an animal doesn't change much; it just looks and acts older. Humans, on the other hand, may have gone through dramatic changes in outlook on life, attitude, career, wisdom, faith, and beliefs—hopefully for the better.

But what is more, human self-determination is not only controlled by rationality but also by morality. Not everything that is thinkable or possible or reasonable is also permissible. Animals, in contrast, do not have any ethical values, so they follow whatever "pops up" in their brains. The relationship between predator and prey, for instance, has nothing to do with morality; if predators really had a conscience guided by morality, their lives would be pretty harsh. Animals never do awful things out of meanness or cruelty, for the simple reason that they have no morality, and thus no cruelty or meanness. But humans definitely have the capacity of performing atrocities. On the other hand, if animals seem to do awful things, it is only because we as human beings consider their actions "awful" according to our standards of morality. Yet we will never arrange court sessions for grizzly bears that maul hikers, because they are not morally responsible for their actions. Since animals have no moral values, they have no duties, no responsibilities, and consequently no rights. If animals had rights, their fellow animals would need to respect those too.

So we are back to this "systematic elusiveness of 'I'" that appears to be so uniquely human. It gives us the wonderful capability of self-reflection, self-awareness, self-transcendence, self-expression, self-determination, introspection, and morality. It changes us into rational and moral beings—beings with a mind and a soul, beings who can make rational and irrational decisions as well as moral and immoral ones. All this should make us aware of the fact that there is a mind behind the brain. Brain surgeons aren't mind surgeons; the mind keeps eluding the knife of the dissecting scientist. Although the brain may give me intelligence, it is the mind that gives me intellect—including rationality and morality.

At this point I need to explain my terminology further. I have been using terms such as "I," "self," "mind," "soul," and even "spirit" interchangeably. I do so because I do not want to go into a difficult debate about how and where they differ; that is outside the scope of this discussion. In this book, I will lump them all together under the term "mind," taken as a non-material, spiritual entity to be at least distinguished from the material entity of the human body. For those who want more distinctions, I would say mind is the intellectual part of "self," of "soul." I would define the mind as the soul's eye, its light—or to put it differently, the mind is the power of the soul by which we can tell true from false and right from wrong. If you take rationality and morality away from us, we are indeed mere animals. If we deny such distinctions and see ourselves as animals, we will find reasons for treating each other as they do!

As noted earlier, even if we come to fully understand the human brain, we will never fully understand the human mind, for it requires a mind to understand the brain and it requires a human subject to study any objects. It requires a subject to make sense of pictures or words, so they become objects of knowledge based on mental concepts; without "I" as a subject, those items remain meaningless. In our knowing, we are indeed more than what we know; we are rational and moral beings—and that is what makes us really tick.

So we end up being very different from our "relatives" in the animal world. Although we are flesh as they are flesh because we breed, feed, bleed, and excrete like they do, we are also very exceptional creatures in this universe. There are things that set us apart from other creatures; that is our rationality and our morality—as I have shown in this Chapter.

Intermission 4A

The Mirror Test

Why do animals lack any form of self-expression? The reason is simple: They have no real "self." Although monkeys are in fact able to use mirror images to locate things and other animals in real space, they have been given months, sometimes years, in which to recognize *themselves* in mirrors. But they typically either neglect their mirror image or treat it as a potential aggressor. Yet it is true that chimpanzees and orangutans like elephants and dolphins (and unlike gorillas), show some capacity of recognizing themselves in a mirror.

Scientists, after marking an animal with a visible as well as a not directly visible dye spot, have been testing whether and how the animal reacts to the visible dye located on its own body while ignoring the control dye. This so-called mirror test was devised in 1970 by psychologist Gordon G. Gallup to detect self-awareness in animals by studying whether an animal can recognize its own reflection in a mirror as an image of itself. Although the mirror test ranks high on the evolutionists' schema, it doesn't entitle them to equate self-recognition with reflection on the self, let alone self-awareness. Why not?

First of all, passing the mirror test is merely evidence of superior neural capabilities; of being arguably based more on face-recognition than a sense of "self." Dogs, on the other hand, perform poorly on the mirror test, but they do seem to be able to recognize their own scent. We are dealing here at least partly with a form of learned behavior. When first exposed to a mirror, most apes react to their reflection as they would to another member of the same species; but eventually they may learn to recognize that their mirror image is a reflection of their own body.

Second, animals have an inherent ability to classify, distinguish, and recognize faces and scents; so why would they not be able to classify a face or scent as coming with one particular body—their own body. The fact that birds, for instance, can clean their own feathers doesn't mean they have the capacity of self-awareness and self-reflection.

Third, the mirror test shows us that some animals can recognize their own body. But that shouldn't surprise us, since animals drinking from water surfaces should be used to seeing a reflection of their own bodies and they won't attack their own image. But do they also have a sense of "self," a sense of past and future, knowing that they exist in a particular time and place? I doubt it, for mirrors mirror a body, but not a self. Animals won't make a trip to the water just to have a look at "themselves" in the "mirror."

Finally, the mirror test may tell us much more about ourselves than about the animal world. When we observe apes recognizing "themselves" in a mirror it connects with our questions about the human self, and our dissimilarity from the animal world. It is exactly because animals have no "self" that they can't follow the golden rule that says, "what you do not want to be done to yourself, do not do that to others."

In other words, even if animals are able to recognize "themselves" in a mirror, they may have some body-recognition, perhaps some self-recognition, but not necessarily self-awareness; and they certainly do not have the human capabilities of self-reflection, self-transcendence, self-expression, self-determination, and morality. Where do these come from? These capabilities are not based on our brain structure, as human brains do not differ much from the brains of apes. And we note that elephants' brains are much larger without greatly increased function. Despite this, for those looking to locate the essence of the human mind in anatomy, it remains tempting to make the mind as measurable and quantifiable as the brain. No wonder that Francis Galton, a cousin of Charles Darwin, was quick to launch "psychometrics" in order to correlate head sizes with mental capacities. But the attempt at correlation failed.

Believing that all mental faculties are represented by different brain areas, the so-called phrenologists of more than a century ago tried to locate and measure such areas, but they failed. The "phrenologists" of today use brain scans to analyze the mind by studying the brain's neuronal network, but they continue to fail.

No, it is not really the brain that sets us apart, not even our DNA, for that is not very different either. Unlike bodily coordination, mental orchestration is not a matter of anatomy, physiology, genes, or brains. The brain is just a material vehicle for an immaterial mind—or to put it explicitly, the mind uses the brain the way a programmer uses a computer. It is this immaterial mind that gives human beings such an endless potential that they can even picture themselves in make-believe situations—never seen, never experienced before. The sky is the limit!

Intermission 4B

Is There a Ghost in the Machine?

Following Plato, the French philosopher René Descartes distinguished "physical substance," *res extensa* which can be measured and divided from *res cogitans*, which is not extended and not cleavable.[1] The body clearly belongs to the former category whereas the mind was viewed by Descartes as something non-physical, as something lacking shape, size, and location. Yet he modeled everything after the grammar of mechanics: as the body is an acting thing, a machine, so is the mind a "thinking thing." In his famous summation, "I think, therefore I am," this "I" was considered a non-physical thing, an "I-thing," existing independently of the physical brain, yet maintaining some kind of causal interaction with the physical connections of nerves and muscles. Descartes thought that perhaps the pineal gland was the interaction point.

But could this "I-thing" be located somewhere in the body? A popular theory that was in vogue for a long time was that the human mind works with something like an "inner observer" or "mental agent"—something like a "man in the machine." While watching a movie, viewers see the images as something separate from themselves projected on the screen. Could we perhaps explain this by supposing that the light from the screen forms images on the retina that are transferred next to the visual cortex, where they are then scanned by an "inner observer" who is located in the brain behind the cortex? Or when people give commands to their body, could it possibly be that some "mental agent" is steering the body like a piano player would play the piano? No, not really. If this theory were correct, we would end up with "an observer in an observer" or "a piano player inside a piano player." You feel it coming—infinite regress!

Sometimes this is called the homunculus (little man) theory— explaining a phenomenon in terms of the very phenomenon that it is

---

[1] René Descartes, *Descartes Discourse on Method and the Meditations*, Trans. F. E. Sutcliff (Penguin Books, 1968), Second Meditation, Part 1.

supposed to explain. I am reminded of "ancient" biologists, such as Hartsoeker in 1694 and Dalempatius in 1699, who thought that through their simple microscopes they could discern a human person inside a human sperm cell.[2] What they thought they saw would entail that this human person in turn would also carry sperm cells with human persons in them, and so on and on. Explaining "man" by assuming "a man in the man-machine" is the same thing. As it turns out, we cannot take the mind as an agent hidden somewhere in the body, or as "a man in the man-machine." The brain does not harbor any detectable agent who plays the "piano" of the body. Yet scientists—and neuroscientists in particular—would like to locate the mind somewhere in the body as a physical entity, hoping that by dissecting the human brain they can dissect the human mind.

Of course, it is well known that parts of the brain "mirror," or represent, certain parts of the body, and since scientists always search for material causes, they have also been searching for a part of the brain that regulates the brain itself. But there can be no such physical brain part in charge of the brain; the brain doesn't have a part that mirrors itself. Once again, the mind is eluding the knife of the dissecting scientist.

The mystery remains, though; we cannot locate any "piano player," yet we do hear his or her "music." Because the mind does not occur on the physical map of the body, it may seem as if it is nowhere in the chain of bodily activities, yet it is the "soul" of it all and pervades the entire body. In contrast to an eye blinking there is a "soul" or an "I" behind an eye winking.

By the way, some philosophers try to explain this enigmatic topic in terms of computer language which may clarify some, but certainly not all, of the implications. First, there is the "hardware," or the machinery of our brain. This hardware includes the material our brain is made of and the physical processes taking place there. Then there is also the non-physical "software," which is the program making the machinery run in a certain way. According to the computer analogy, our mind is *something* like the programming software, not to be confused with the machinery itself. Needless to

---

[2] Nicolaas Hartsoeker (1656 -1725) Dutch mathematician and physicist.
François de Plantade, under the assumed name Dalempatius (1670-1741) French astronomer.

say, if the machinery is broken the software can't perform well. But just as it is nonsense to ask how a computer program causes the computer circuits to solve mathematical equations, so it does not make sense to ask how non-physical thoughts make the brain perform certain physical reactions.

No matter how attractive the computer analogy may be to understanding the working of the brain, it does not help us to understand the working of the mind. Note the difference in the tasks performed by the computer and the human brain. When computers perform tasks such as providing information in word processors, spreadsheet tools and other applications, the mind of a human subject is crucial for interpreting the computer information as being some kind of code with a specific meaning.

Without the mind of a human subject, things do not have any meaning or make any sense until they become objects of knowledge. So computers cannot explain, but can only presume, the human mind. As I said earlier, computers do not create thoughts, but they may carry thoughts once they are created by the human mind. The mind uses the brain as the programmer uses the computer. The mind may look "spooky," but we cannot do without it. So the mystery remains!

Chapter 5

What Ought to Be Done

Each time I hear of demonstrations or protests in the news, I realize again that we are not just matter-of-fact creatures. People who participate in the demonstrations are not telling us what is the case but what *ought* to be the case. Their banners and boards are not stating facts, such as "1+1=2" or "E=mc^2." No, they express that the people protesting are pro-life, anti-abortion, pro-choice, anti-war, anti-racism, anti-death-penalty, or for some other moral course of action. The protesters want to tell us what is morally right or wrong and what ought to be done in life. These are situations where rationality calls for morality: not all that is rationally possible is morally permissible.

It cannot be denied that people consider certain actions morally right or wrong and therefore ought or ought not to be done. Even little children know what is fair or not fair when they are playing games. The fact that we have "standards" for judging human actions cannot be denied. Not only do we observe things, events, and actions, but we also *evaluate* them by saying they were right, or admitting they were wrong and should have been done differently.

I realize this doesn't mean that the standards we use to evaluate actions are therefore valid and correct. That is an altogether different issue, which we will discuss later. When we evaluate things, we discern a specific feature or property that turns them into something valuable—which is called a value. Although there are different kinds of values, such as moral, aesthetic, and religious, it is the moral values that are best known. Moral values summon us to action, to what ought to be done in life.

If you ask me what it means for something to be called "good" or "wrong," I would respond that we need to make an important distinction first. Something can be "good" in relation to a given goal or objective. Medical rules, for instance, are "good" for the purpose of medical care. I prefer to call them rules, norms, or standards rather than values. Some people, though, call them instrumental values.

That is all right, of course, but what remains true is that these values are relative values because they tell us what we need to do in order to attain something else. If anyone ever wonders why a certain act is "good" in this instrumental sense, we can provide an explanation in terms of its objective. By a simple yes or no does the act meet its objective? If it does, it is considered "good." And every action that does not meet the objective is consequently "wrong." But I emphasize that this doesn't mean that those actions are also right or wrong in a moral sense.

In a moral context, "good" has a very different meaning. Whatever is called "good" in a moral sense tells us what we ought to do—no matter what, whether we like it or not, whether we feel it or not, or whether we want it or not. Only in this case would we speak of moral values. Moral values are absolute, because they tell us what we ought to do as human beings, irrespective of any other objective. Hence they are generally called intrinsic values. They make for universal, absolute, objective, and binding prescriptions; they are ends-in-themselves, and are not like instrumental rules, means-to-other-ends. In other words, there's nothing "useful" about them. If anyone ever wonders why a certain act such as saving a human life is "good" in this moral sense, we have no explanation to offer and cannot refer to other ends; all we can say is "it is self-evident." The "moral eye" sees values in life, just like the "physical eye" sees colors in nature. Moral values are definitely real, but obviously not so in a physical sense.

It has been suggested that moral values are "evident" because they are grounded in our genes—another example of "nothing-buttery." If that were so, we wouldn't be morally obligated, but we would only feel obligated; our genetic make-up would only have us *believe* that our moral obligations rest on an objective foundation. This would, so to speak, make for a collective illusion, foisted on us by our genes. But it seems to me that such a foundation would be as fragile as the genetic material it is said to be made of—DNA.

If this view that moral values are grounded in our genes were right, morality could still be something very "real," but it would be without a solid basis; it would not have the universality that is supposed to transcend differences in culture, era, and personal preferences. As a result, moral values would indeed seem as if they were evident, but would in effect be worth nothing. They would be resting on quicksand. Their intrinsic value would be like what some people call the "intrinsic value" of gold; gold has no value in itself, but gets its value from us, because we highly value its properties.

Yet some biologists and philosophers propose that evolutionary biology can explain how humanity acquired its morality. Their "magic wand" is the theory of natural selection. The logic behind their position is: Since it seems to be an important job of cognition to make rational and moral decisions, our cognitive capacities must have been shaped by evolutionary pressures and therefore bear the stamp of our long evolutionary history. The better the predictive capacities, the better are the organism's chances for survival.[1] As a consequence, moral actions would not be right or wrong, but only successful or not in terms of survival.

Take the example of incest. There is an almost universal human taboo on incest—phrased as a moral law, it says, "intercourse with very close relatives is wrong and hence forbidden." Well, these biologists would point out that inbreeding between close relatives tends to bring out recessive lethal traits and other afflictions that lessen the offspring's reproductive success. Hence they argue that natural selection has been promoting a genetic basis for behavioral avoidance of intercourse with close relatives, and that is where they believe this moral value stems from. If this were so, the *moral* value would definitely be on its way out.

Or think of moral laws given in the Fifth and Sixth Commandments of the Decalogue: "You shall not kill" and "You shall not commit adultery." Some biologists have made the case that humans must be monogamous "by nature," just like swans and some other animals, since that would give the offspring a better protection and that is why natural selection must have promoted monogamy— making a biological basis of the Sixth Commandment. Others have made the assertion that killing members of the same species would undermine the persistence of the species, and consequently the prohibition was selected by the process of natural selection. They even consider the moral value of paternal care for children as a product of natural selection; their reasoning is that fathers who do not feel an "instinctive" responsibility toward their underage children would reduce their offspring's reproductive success. What all

---

[1] See, for instance, Patricia Smith Churchland, *Brain-Wise: Studies in Neurophilosophy* (Cambridge, MA: MIT Press, 2002).

these cases have in common is that morality is supposedly based on genes promoted by natural selection. They tell you that there is nothing *moral* about moral values but that they are just inborn!

What is wrong with such a viewpoint? My fundamental objection is as follows: Why would we need an articulated moral rule to reinforce what by nature we would or would not desire to do anyway? Reality tells us that far too many people are willing to break a moral rule when they can get away with it! Too many parents ignore their so-called "natural" responsibility. Too many spouses violate the Sixth Commandment, "You shall not commit adultery." Too many people also violate the Fifth Commandment, "You shall not kill." Are these people really going against their genes?

My conclusion is that, apparently, moral laws tell us to do what our genes do *not* make us do by nature. Morality is about something that is outside the scope of biology, actually beyond the reach of science. Of course, it shouldn't have taken us by surprise that morality cannot be established through biology, as biology is just not a know-all or cure-all. Biology is blind to moral values, so it cannot possibly discern anything that is on its "blind spot." Science cannot control morality, but morality must control science instead.

The question remains, where does morality come from if it is not rooted in our biology, our physiology, our genes, or our DNA? If biology cannot explain morality, what else can? Many people have tried to base morality and its values on something that is not moral in itself. One of the most popular explanations of this kind is given by utilitarianism; it considers something morally right depending on its effects—that is, if it leads to "the greater happiness of a greater number of people." The problem here is that we would treat moral values, which as I said earlier are intrinsic values, as if they were instrumental values. That is, relative values which tell us what we need to do in order to attain something else, such as greater happiness. The problem with utilitarianism is that it considers as morally right those acts instrumental to some kind of happiness. However, moral values are not instrumental values but intrinsic values; they are ends-in-themselves, not means-to-other-ends.

You probably wonder how moral values could ever qualify as ends-in-themselves and entities of their own. Let me explain this point with an example used by President Abraham Lincoln. In his words:

If A. can prove, however conclusively, that he may, of right, enslave B.—why may not B. snatch the same argument, and prove equally, that he may enslave A.?—You say A. is white, and B. is black. It is color, then; the lighter, having the right to enslave the darker? Take care. By this rule, you are to be slave to the first man you meet, with a fairer skin than your own. You mean the whites are intellectually the superiors of the blacks; and, therefore have the right to enslave them? Take care again. By this rule, you are to be slave to the first man you meet, with an intellect superior to your own." [2]

I would say that Honest Abe's example is truly powerful. His point is clear: all the answers you might come up with to defend your moral claim actually use non-moral or morally irrelevant criteria. And the same holds for the value of human life, which cannot be based on biological standards, since those are by definition morally irrelevant. Moral values are ends-in-themselves—not disposable means-to-other-ends. In morality, there's no "Thou shall not...unless..."

A similar point has been made by other thinkers. The British philosopher G. E. Moore spoke of the naturalistic fallacy.[3] This consists of erroneously reducing a moral property (being good or right) to a natural property (being natural, functional, genetic, more evolved, better for the majority, or whatever). Therefore it would be a fallacy to define moral notions in non-moral terms. Science discovers the way things are, not the way they ought to be. The fact that something *is* this way doesn't mean that it *ought to be* this way. The fact that something is natural doesn't imply that it is also a moral value that ought to be enforced. The fact that various human beings are genetically different doesn't imply that we ought to value them differently. The fact that natural selection is "natural" doesn't mean that it also should be put into action as a moral duty. Or in line with the naturalistic fallacy: if slavery, murder, prostitution, or what have you helps us fit into our environment in line with the dogma of "survival of the fittest," there wouldn't be anything morally wrong with any of those. But we all know better, don't we!

---

[2] Abraham Lincoln, *His Speeches and Writings*, ed. Roy P. Basler (Cambridge, MA: Da Capo Press, 2001), 278.

[3] G. E. Moore [1903], *Principia Ethica* (Cambridge University Press, 1993).

So we must come to the conclusion that morality can't be based on anything non-moral. It is not rooted in our genes, it is not the product of natural selection, it is not the result of any legislation, it is not a scientific conclusion, and it is not based on anything useful or beneficial such as "the greater happiness of a greater number of people." All of these substitutes are morally irrelevant, since morality includes a new dimension that only morality has access to. Because of its absolute values, morality cannot be based on anything that is relative or non-moral by nature. In short, there is just nothing "useful" about morality.

But that makes the following question even more pressing: if morality can never be based on other ends, where do moral values come from? How can we prove them to be right? Earlier I said that they are self-evident. If you were to ask me why it is forbidden to kill someone I would not have much to say and could not refer to something else, other than the Fifth Commandment. Claiming that the act of killing is wrong cannot be substantiated by anything else, for that would make for an instrumental value. We just find it evident that killing human beings is wrong. The "moral eye" sees moral values in life, just like the "physical eye" sees physical colors in nature. Moral values and the natural laws of morality belong to the "unseen" world we discussed earlier; they are immaterial and yet very real. We didn't invent them, but discovered them. They do not just exist in our minds.

That *sounds* nice, you might counter, but moral values keep changing over time and between cultures. So there goes their self-evident existence, doesn't it? Not really! It is not the moral values themselves that change over time, but it is our moral evaluations that may change. Evaluations are subjective, whereas values are objective. Moral evaluations are our personal feelings or discernments regarding moral values.

Evaluations concern someone's personal attitude toward moral values, causing some to think that morality is determined by special-interest groups or a majority vote. Although some people maintain that "having value" is the same as "being valued," the value itself (being a value) should be distinguished from human attitudes toward values (being valued). People who deny this distinction believe that, in making evaluations, we create values in accordance with these evaluations. So when evaluations change, the moral values and laws are believed to change as well. If that were so, evaluations—and thus values—would be a matter of utter relativity, depending on the era, culture, and location of the person who makes the evaluations.

I would point out that we have utter confusion unless absolute, objective values are different from relative, subjective evaluations. But then you may question how we could ever have access to those absolute and universal values if our evaluations keep changing. No wonder that such thinking has led many to accept what they call "moral relativism." This asserts that the values themselves are subject to change during the course of human history—ruled by a majority vote, so to speak. This viewpoint of relativists amounts to an *absolute* claim stating that there are no absolutes (except for this absolute claim itself, of course). Relativists reject any authority, but want to be the new authority!

There are compelling reasons for taking the side of moral absolutists who emphasize that evaluations are merely a reflection of the way we discern moral values and react to them at the current time. In other words, evaluations may change, but values won't. Absolutists want to stress that moral values and laws are eternal, objective, and absolute. While relativists wouldn't acknowledge the possibility of making moral mistakes, absolutists would. As a matter of fact, the absolutists' view is more common than you might think. Even in science our current understanding of mathematical and physical laws constantly needs revision until we reach a better understanding of those laws the way they really are. In a similar way, we assume that there are absolute and universal laws of nature, although we may not yet have fully captured them.

So is there a way to justify values and laws in morality? Again, the only apt answer is: "They are just (self-) evident," but their evidence is not of an empirical and material nature. Some among us are able to clearly discern certain values and evaluate them properly, whereas others are not able to. Anyone who does not see their evidence must be "blind." Just as there are color-blind people, there are also value-blind people. The "natural law" of morality can be discovered by everyone, whether religious or not, who is not value-blind. It enables us to discern by reason the good and the evil, the truth and the lie. Thomas Aquinas describes the natural law as "the light of understanding placed in us by God; through it we know what we must

WHAT MAKES YOU TICK?

do and what we must avoid."[4] It is the natural law that is our ultimate moral authority. Its principal precepts are expressed in the Ten Commandments. President Ronald Reagan used to say, "I have wondered at times about what the Ten Commandments would have looked like if Moses had run them through the U.S. Congress..."[5] Moral evaluations may be based on a majority vote, but moral values are not.[6]

Let me illustrate this point a little further. A few centuries ago, slavery was not generally evaluated as morally wrong, but nowadays it is considered morally wrong by most people. Did our moral values change? No, they did not, but our evaluations certainly did. Only a few people in the past were able to discern the objective and universal value of personal freedom and human rights versus slavery, whereas most of their contemporaries were blind to this value. How often were the best people who had the clearest discernment of moral values persecuted by the mass of blind people! And yet the advancement of humanity did often depend on these very people having a sharper and better discernment of moral values. It is not the values that change in the course of human evolution but their evaluations—that is, our subjective attitudes toward these objective values. Anyone who does not see their evidence is blind.

But the question remains: where do these universal standards come from? There is no other way than acknowledging that moral values have an extra dimension and therefore must be derived from a different realm—from the "Grand Beyond." We are in fact standing at its gates!

---

[4] Thomas Aquinas, *Dec. praec.* I.

[5] Quoted in Matthew N. Beckmann, *Pushing the Agenda* (Cambridge University Press, 2010), 1.

[6] Just for the record, there may be moral laws other than the "natural law" that only religious people know about.

Intermission 5A

Human Dignity

Many people think that human rights are closely connected with human dignity. In one sense it must be agreed that they are indeed closely connected; in another sense it must be denied since it depends on how rights and dignity are defined.

The idea of human dignity is not a new concept, but is originally a Judeo-Christian concept. It got a fresh look after World War II when the first photographs of inhumane atrocities in the Nazi concentration camps appeared. So in 1948, the United Nations (UN) affirmed in the Universal Declaration of Human Rights that "all human beings are born free and equal in dignity and rights."[1]

However, the UN assumed a general understanding of "human dignity" but didn't define it. As a result, the Declaration of Human Rights was placed at the mercy of special-interest groups, who endeavor to establish new sexual and reproductive "rights," such as abortion, and the new "rights" of scientists to experiment with human embryos, as well as another invention, the "last civil right"— to die. Obviously, the concept of human dignity has become what Adam Schulman called "a placeholder for whatever it is about human beings that entitles them to basic human rights and freedoms."[2] It has become a placeholder for a human-made morality. Most of these "new rights" are not really moral rights but rather legal entitlements. We have a clear case here of word inflation. Human rights are not man made entitlements but God-given rights that we cannot invent on our own. A right is a moral concept based on a moral law, whereas an entitlement is a legal (and not necessarily moral) notion based on a

---

[1] UN General Assembly, *Universal Declaration of Human Rights*, 10 December 1948, 217 A (III), available at: http://www.unhcr.org/refworld/docid/3ae6b3712c.html.

[2] Edmund D. Pellegrino, Adam Schulman, and Thomas W. Merrill, eds., *Human Dignity and Bioethics: Essays Commissioned by the President's Council on Bioethics* (Notre Dame, IN: University of Notre Dame Press, 2009), Chap.1.

legal law. There are no minority rights or sexual and reproductive rights; these are, at most, entitlements.

And what about animal rights? Animals have no morality, so they can follow whatever "pops up" in their brains. The relationship between predator and prey, for instance, has nothing to do with morality; if predators really had a conscience guided by morality, their lives would be pretty tough. Since animals have no moral values, they have no duties, no responsibilities, and consequently no rights. If animals had rights, their fellow animals would also need to respect those. Dogs may act as if they are "caring," but they just follow their instinct. Dogs happen to have such an instinct, whereas cats lack it, as it is not in their genes.

Humans, on the other hand, do have moral values. That is why they have to treat animals, God's other creatures, humanely and responsibly—not because animals deserve it, but because humans owe it to their Maker and to themselves, being stewards of what the Maker created.

Intermission 5B

Is There Altruism in the Animal World?

Evolutionists like to explain everything with the theory of natural selection. They have even attempted to infiltrate the domain of morality, including its concept of altruism. You might think altruism would be safe against the attacks of evolutionists because altruism goes against the very idea of natural selection. Altruism is considered to be unselfish behavior—a sacrifice of personal comfort for the benefit of others—whereas natural selection is based on the principle of increasing one's own reproductive success at the expense of others. They can't go together, can they?

Indeed, at first sight altruism seems to be a problem in relation to natural selection. But socio-biologists such as E. O. Wilson did find a biological explanation.[1] The pressing question in socio-biology is the following: how can altruistic behavior in the animal world still be advantageous to its agent? Well, socio-biologists did come up with some answers, which I won't discuss in detail. By introducing some clear distinctions I hope to gain a better understanding of the confusions we could come across in this discussion.

First of all, we have the biological version of altruism—which I call bio-altruism. In the animal world, we do indeed find many examples of animals helping one another; just think of sterile worker bees "unselfishly" helping the queen raise her own progeny. Socio-biologists would explain bio-altruism as a form of helping one's close relatives, because these carry DNA very similar to one's own. Since natural selection is a matter of balancing the benefits against the costs, bio-altruism is a way of promoting one's "own" DNA by diminishing one's own offspring (a cost) but increasing the offspring of one's relatives (a benefit). And that is exactly what bees

---

[1] E. O. Wilson, *Sociobiology: The New Synthesis* (Cambridge MA: Harvard University Press, Twenty-fifth Anniversary Edition, 1975/2000).

accomplish. Because these Hymenoptera have a very peculiar sexual system, females are more closely related to sisters (sharing 75 percent of their genetic material) than to daughters (sharing only 50 percent). So sterile females actually increase their own reproductive success by 25 percent in an "indirect" way—by helping rear their queen-sister's progeny (75 percent) rather than their own (50 percent).

This approach has many more applications in biology than you might think. As the geneticist J. B. S. Haldane once said, "I will lay down my life for two brothers or eight cousins." His calculation of costs and benefits was based on the fact that in a regular sexual system, siblings share half of their genetic material, whereas cousins only share one-eight. By helping close relatives, one is somehow promoting the dispersal of one's own genetic material, but in an indirect way through the relatives. For humans one's genetic material could be equally advanced through two brothers or eight cousins since:

$$8 \times \frac{1}{8} = 2 \times \frac{1}{2} = 1$$

That is what I call bio-altruism.

Secondly, there is also a sociological version of altruism—which I call socio-altruism. It is based on the principle of helping those who return the help. I give, so you give! Divided you may fall, but united you may conquer! This happens, for example, when two or more organisms, such as chimpanzees, band together and in helping others, help themselves. Socio-biologists have studied this phenomenon with game theory, and they have been rather successful doing so. I would say this is a success for socio-biology. And let us leave it at that.

Socio-biology may have solved the problems of bio-altruism and socio-altruism, but has it also solved the problem of altruism in ethics—what I call moral-altruism? Moral-altruism is a moral concept that is altogether different from bio-altruism and socio-altruism. As will be seen, the answer is definitely no:

> Bio-altruism is behavior with the *effect* that one's own offspring is diminished but compensated for by helping relatives. So it may be functional and advantageous at times.
> Socio-altruism is behavior with the *motive* of helping others, but limited to those who return the help. In helping others, one

helps oneself according to the Roman motto *Do ut des* (I give so that you will give).

Moral-altruism is behavior for the sake of the *value* of serving others, without expecting any advantage. This is what we really and rightly call "unselfish altruism."

We need some clear terminology here. What you *ought* to achieve (which is a moral value) is not necessarily what you *want* to achieve (which is a motive or intention). And what you want to achieve is not always what you actually *do* achieve (which is an effect). Let us remain clear-headed and not mix them up.

As we discovered earlier, biology, or one of its branches, sociobiology, cannot have a monopolistic claim on human behavior, because biology will never be able to tell us a comprehensive, all-inclusive story about human life and human behavior. Since moral values add their own, new dimension and perspective to our world, there is not much hope for those numerous efforts of fully converting moral behavior into a non-moral phenomenon. Science has no access to morality!

Chapter 6

Help from Beyond

It is very unusual to see a cow eating fruit from a tree. But I saw it once. It is very unusual because it is awfully hard for cows—used to looking down to the grass they are eating—to look up to food hanging above them in the trees. C. S. Lewis put this in more general terms: "As long as you are looking down, you cannot see something that is above you."[1] So far we have as a rule been looking down—"down" to the "lower" levels of DNA, genes, neurons, brains, computers, and such. But ultimately, those elementary levels are not enough to make us "tick." The words we quoted earlier were prophetic: "Genes can't possibly explain all of what makes us what we are." Craig Venter of Celera Genomics, whom I quoted earlier, may not have intended as I do that much of what we are is also determined by rationality and morality. But take rationality and morality away and we are back to where we came from—mere animals.

So let us try to look "up" for a change: You and I have minds endowed with rationality and morality; we are human beings who can make rational and moral decisions, and that, of course, also entails that we can make irrational and immoral decisions. But where do rationality and morality come from? The answer must go like this: not from "below" but from "above"; they do not come from DNA, but from where DNA came from; they are not part of physics but of metaphysics. And yet they make us "tick."

Let us start with rationality. Rationality is not a matter of intelligence but of intellect. Rationality is our capacity for abstract reasoning and having reasons for our thoughts, thus giving us access to the "unseen" world of thoughts, laws, and truths—allowing us to be masters of our own actions. Reasoning is pondering realities beyond what we experience through our senses.

---

[1] C. S. Lewis, *Mere Christianity,* Third edition (San Francisco: Harper, 2001), 74.

Animals, for their part, seem to live their lives entirely in the present, without having any thoughts about the past or the future. If animals have a pedigree, it is thanks to their owners; if they have birthdays, wish lists, appointments, or schedules, it is because their owners create those; and if they have graves, those were dug by their owners as well. Have you ever seen animals dressing themselves or training other animals or keeping them as their pets? What a disparity! Only humans are able to keep pets and train them. Only humans can complain that they felt treated like animals. Only humans are conscious of time; they can study the past, recognize the present, and anticipate the future; they even desire to transcend time, thinking about living forever. Only humans make rational decisions. Only humans know about what is "above." Only humans wonder "what caused, or will cause, what, and why?" Only human beings have inquisitive minds asking questions such as "Where do we come from?" They are always in search of some kind of worldview or explanation of life—that certainly goes far beyond their need for food. You may consider philosophy a pretty sophisticated enterprise, but there probably isn't one human being who doesn't philosophize; each one of us is destined to start philosophizing at some point in life. Reading this book is, hopefully, one of those moments!

As a matter of fact, it is rationality that makes us ask profound philosophical questions such as: why there is something rather than nothing? Or more specifically: why this world is comprehensible? As Albert Einstein has said, the most incomprehensible thing, the greatest mystery about this world, is that it is comprehensible.[2] If it were not, science would be impossible. Another pertinent question would be this: why is this world so orderly instead of being completely chaotic? If there were no order in the universe, it wouldn't make sense to search for laws of nature in physics, chemistry, biology, and other disciplines. Or consider these questions: why do like causes have like effects, and why does the future depend on the past? If that were not the case, we could never explain or

---

[2] Quoted by Antonina Vallentin, *Einstein: A Biography* (London: Weidenfeld and Nicolson, 1954), 24, quoted as from Einstein's article "Physics and Reality" *Journal of the Franklin Institute* (March 1936). However, in the actual article, reprinted in *Out of My Later Years* (New York: Gramercy Publishing, 1993), the quote is: "One may say 'the eternal mystery of the world is its comprehensibility.' "

predict anything; there wouldn't even be such a thing as falsification, for the fact that scientific evidence can either support or refute a scientific hypothesis is possible only if there is order in this universe. Without order, there wouldn't be any falsifying evidence. As rational beings, we want a rational answer to the above questions.

The issue at stake can be worded as follows: why does the rationality as present in our minds correspond with the rationality present in the world? A rational answer would be that their congruence can best be explained at a deeper, or higher, level: the Rationality of a Creator who respects reason. That would be Leibniz' principle of sufficient reason in reply to Newton's question "Whence arise all the Order and Beauty that we see in the World?"[3]

Arguably the best rational answer would go along the following lines, phrased in the form of rhetorical questions:

- Could nature be intelligible if it were not created by an intelligent Creator?

- Could there be order in this world if there were no orderly Creator?

- Could there be scientific laws if there were no rational Lawgiver?

- Could there be moral laws if there were no moral Lawgiver?

- Could there be design in nature if there were no intelligent Designer?

- Could there be human minds if there were no Divine Mind?

I would say the answer to all the above questions is "No," unless you are prepared to give up on rationality. The answer that things just are the way they are is not a very satisfying response; our universe need not be the way it is, and it need not even exist. In other words, our universe is neither necessary nor absolute, but finite and dependent instead; the more philosophical term is *contingent*. However, if there is no inherent necessity for the universe to exist, then the universe is not self-explaining and therefore must find an explanation outside itself. Obviously it cannot be grounded in something else that is also finite and not self-explaining, for that

---

[3] R.S. Westfall, *Never at Rest* (Cambridge University Press, 1980), 647.

would lead to vicious infinite regress. Therefore it can derive only from an unconditioned, infinite, and ultimate ground, which is a Creator God. As a theologian put it, "Has God not therefore created the world 'in himself,' giving it time in his eternity, finitude in his infinity, space in his omnipresence, and freedom in his selfless love?"[4]

Without the notion of the universe as a created entity, even science would be a shaky, problematic, and irrational enterprise. But you might object: isn't the concept of creation in itself also a shaky concept? You could argue, for instance, that the Big Bang Theory has replaced what we call creation. Some cosmologists have indeed fallen into this trap. The physicist Stephen Hawking, for instance, even went as far as to say that the universe created itself from nothing, which he calls "spontaneous creation":

> Because there is a law such as gravity, the universe can and will create itself from nothing. Spontaneous creation is the reason there is something rather than nothing.[5]

No wonder this made the physicist Carl Sagan exclaim, in the preface of one of Hawking's books, that such a cosmological model "left nothing for a creator to do."[6] Others, such as the cosmologist Lee Smolin, made sure there is no space left for a Creator by saying "by definition the universe is all there is, and there can be nothing outside it."[7]

The objection to the idea of spontaneous creation is that it is sheer philosophical nonsense; for something to create itself, it would have to exist before it came into existence—which is logically impossible. How could the universe "create" itself from nothing—let alone cause itself? A cause cannot just cause itself; it would have to exist before it came into existence. "Nothingness" is a highly unusual kind of stuff that is more difficult to observe than other things! It is not a thing, but the absence of anything.

---

[4] Jürgen Moltmann, *The Trinity and the Kingdom of God* (London: SCM Press, 1981), 109.

[5] Stephen Hawking and Leonard Mlodinow, *The Grand Design* (New York: Random House, Bantam Books, 2010), 180.

[6] Stephen Hawking, *A Brief History of Time* (New York, Bantam Books, 1988), x.

[7] Lee Smolin, *Three Roads to Quantum Gravity* (New York: Basic Books, 2001), 17.

When Hawking tells us that gravity would be able to create the universe, I would argue that the law of gravity would have to exist before there was gravity. Such a law is not something just residing in our minds, but "it is out there" for us to discover. Isn't it amazing how good physicists can be such poor philosophers? Albert Einstein hit the nail right on the head when he said: "the man of science is a poor philosopher."[8] The physical chemist Peter Atkins has the overconfidence to state that "there is hope for a scientific elucidation of creation from nothing."[9] Previously he had said that science has limitless power and must even be able to account for the "emergence of everything from absolutely nothing."[10]

What is behind all these philosophical errors? Scientists speak about the beginning of the universe usually in terms of the Big Bang, and they may think they are also referring to the *creation* of the universe. However, the concepts of "creation" and "Big Bang" are very different from each other: creation isn't some trigger event like the Big Bang.

In fact, creation isn't an event at all. On the contrary, creation must come "first" before any events, even a Big Bang, that follow. The CERN laboratory for high energy physics and its famous Large Hadron Collider may help unravel the "mystery" of the beginning of this universe, but not the mystery of the creation of this universe. These are two very different kinds of mystery. The Big Bang is very different from the creation "out of nothing." Science is about producing something from something else, whereas creation is about creating something from nothing. That is an old, solid distinction that Thomas Aquinas already made centuries ago.[11] Science is about changes in this universe, but creation is not a change; it is not a change from "nothing" to "something." Creation has everything to do with the philosophical and theological question as to why things exist at all,

---

[8] Albert Einstein, *Out of My Later Years* (New York: Philosophical Library, 1950), 58.

[9] Peter Atkins, *On Being* (Oxford: Oxford University Press, 2011), 12.

[10] Peter Atkins, "The Limitless Power of Science," in *Nature's Imagination: The Frontiers of Scientific Vision*, ed. John Cornwell and Freeman Dyson (Oxford: Oxford University Press, 1995), 131.

[11] Thomas Aquinas, *De Symbolo Apostolorum*, 33.

before they can even change. Creation—but not the Big Bang—is the reason why there is something rather than nothing.

In other words, creation is not about the beginning of this world, but it is about the origin, the ground, and the foundation of this universe, including its beginning and all its subsequent stages. Creation doesn't start things at the beginning of time but keeps them in existence at all times. Thomas Aquinas actually denies that creation is some chronological episode, located somewhere back in time, when he says, "God brought into being both the creature and time together"[12] and "Before the world, there was no time."[13] The first chapter in the Book of Genesis—the creation account—is not about what happened *at* the beginning, but about what everything is based on to begin with—that is, *in* the beginning. Consequently, Genesis is not a scientific theory of the world's beginning, but rather a monotheistic creed about the world's origin and foundation.

So it should be noted the world may have a beginning and a timeline, but creation itself doesn't have a beginning or a timeline; creation actually makes the beginning of the world and its timeline possible. Creation creates chronology, but it is not a part of chronology. Therefore, creation is not a "one-time deal," but it deals with the question of where this world comes from; it doesn't come from the Big Bang, but may have started with the Big Bang. Without creation, there couldn't be a Big Bang, or any evolution at all. Creation sets the "stage" for these and keeps this world in existence. The "rest of the story" would be something for science to tell. Creation creates something from nothing, whereas evolution produces something from something else.

Our contingent reality points to and depends on a non-contingent Reality, an Absolute entity; without the Infinite, nothing finite could even exist. In the words of Isaac Newton:

> The marvelous arrangement and harmony of the universe can only have been accomplished according to the plan of an almighty being.[14]

---

[12] Thomas Aquinas, *Contra Gentiles* II, 32.

[13] Thomas Aquinas, *De Potentia Dei* 3, 2.

[14] We find this common conviction of a harmonious universe already early in the history of science: Johannes Kepler (in his book *Harmonices Mundi*) as

Science can account only for incomplete causes of what exists, whereas creation offers us the complete cause of what exists. Thomas Aquinas calls the former causes secondary causes, whereas the latter cause is a Primary Cause. The Primary Cause is not a cause among other causes, but it causes creatures to be secondary causes. Without a Primary Cause, there couldn't be any of the secondary causes that science deals with.

But there is more to it: without a Creator, we would no longer have any reason for trusting rationality or any scientific reasoning. Why? There is certainly no scientific proof for the fact that the universe is comprehensible and orderly, for science must *assume* that the cosmos is comprehensible and orderly before science can start working. Scientists just assume and trust that nature is in essence law-abiding and comprehensible; they take the world, although perhaps unknowingly, as something created according to an intelligible plan accessible to the human intellect through the natural light of reason. Order and comprehensibility are proto-scientific, which means that these assumptions must come first before science can even begin. No wonder they are called objective, absolute, and universal suppositions. Without such assumptions, we would lose our reason for reasoning and for trusting our own rationality. We would not be able to distinguish "true" from "false." We would have no other rational measures left but ourselves—and that is extremely "thin air."

But where do such assumptions come from—or, put more generally, where does rationality come from? Unlike intelligence, rationality, so we found out, is not rooted in our genes, in our brains, in our anatomy or physiology. It stems from the "Grand Beyond" and does not come from "below" but from "above." In other words, it was "given" to us, not as a product of evolution, but a gift of creation.

Interestingly enough, there is growing evidence that the "scientific revolution" in the fifteenth and sixteenth centuries had its roots more in the Christian Middle Ages than in the world of ancient

---

well as Isaac Newton spoke of the "harmony of the universe." Robert Boyle would call it the "grand economy of the universe" (*Micrographia*, 16). Later on, Albert Einstein would still speak of "the harmony of the Universe." which we try to formulate as 'laws of nature'." (Letter to A. Chapple, February 23, 1954).

Greeks such as Aristotle and of Islamic scholars such as Avicenna.[15] The latter may have been masters in geometry and mathematics, where pure reason reigns, but this made them think they could generate scientific results deductively from passive observation, which would make those conclusions seem logically necessary. It can be seen that the Greek and Muslim traditions of logic and mathematics provided the tools that science would badly need in order to make its ascent, but don't confuse these tools with science itself. There was a different environment needed for applying these tools in a scientific context—and that environment was the Judeo-Christian concept of Creation and a Creator God.

Because the Judeo-Christian God is a reliable God—not confined inside the Aristotelian box, not capricious like the Olympians in ancient Greece, and not entirely beyond human comprehension like in Islam—the world depends on the laws that God has laid down in creation. That is where the order of the universe ultimately comes from. And the only way to find out what this order looks like is to "interrogate" the universe by investigation, exploration, and experiment. Apparently science was born in a Judeo-Christian cradle and is still living off Judeo-Christian capital. Even the nuclear physicist J. Robert Oppenheimer, who was not a Christian, was ready to acknowledge this very fact when he said, "Christianity was needed to give birth to modern science."[16]

One could reasonably claim that the scientific project and its scientific method are an invention of the Catholic Church.[17] It was during the High Middle Ages that many of the great European universities were founded by the Church. One of the first scientists, Bishop Robert Grosseteste, introduced the scientific method, including the concept of falsification, as early as the thirteenth

---

[15] See, for instance, James Hannam, *The Genesis of Science* (Washington, DC: Regnery Publishing, 2011).

[16] J. Robert Oppenheimer, "On Science and Culture," *Encounter* 19, 4 (1962): 3–10.

[17] Scott Locklin, "No Catholic Church, No Scientific Method", *New Oxford Review*, Oct. 2011: 41-43.

century.[18] The Franciscan friar Roger Bacon established concepts such as using hypotheses, experimentation, and verification, so science would be free from foreign authorities and habitual bias. In other words, what some consider a period of darkness was actually a blaze of the light of reason.

What we discovered about rationality seems to hold for morality as well. When asking the question "Where do our absolute moral values come from?" I do not see any other rational answer than this: moral values come directly from "Above." They are God-given. As we found out earlier, morality is not rooted in our genes, it is not the product of natural selection, it is not the result of any legislation, it is not a scientific conclusion, and it is not based on anything useful or beneficial such as the utilitarian "the greater happiness of a greater number of people." All these substitutes are non-moral and completely irrelevant in moral terms, since morality includes a new dimension that only morality has access to. And that is where we need "divine help."

Since morality has got to be from "Above," how could there be moral laws if there were no moral Lawgiver? Morality is somehow "written" in our hearts and minds, guiding us to make the right choices in life. Even little children know that it is not "fair" when someone cheats, because they were born with a moral compass, pointing not to the magnetic north but to the "Above"—to a place where everything is "fair" and where justice reigns and moral values reside. "Above" is the world of what is "unseen" and "invisible."

This conclusion may strike you by surprise, but it is backed by many famous philosophers with various, even unexpected, backgrounds. An atheistic philosopher such as Jean Paul Sartre, for instance, put it in no uncertain terms: if atheism is true, there can be no absolute or objective standard of right and wrong, for there is no eternal heaven that would make values objective and universal. Stated in reverse, there has got to be an eternal heaven for our moral values so as to make them objective and universal. Somehow we need standards "from above" to be moral human beings. Indeed, if there is a Creator, we would not only have a rational lawgiver, who

---

[18] At the end of the first millennium, Pope Sylvester II had already used advanced instruments of astronomical observation, in his passion for understanding the order of the universe.

guarantees order, intelligibility, and predictability, but also a moral lawgiver who guarantees decency, integrity, responsibility, justice, natural moral law, and human rights.

It was Friedrich Nietzsche, who of all philosophers might be expected to devalue religion, who clearly understood how devastating the decline of religion has been to the ethics of society. If we are only the fortuitous effects of physical causes, we have no other moral measures but ourselves. That is why Nietzsche could say that humanism and other "moral" ideologies shelter themselves in caves and venerate shadows of the God they once believed in; they are holding something they can't provide themselves, mere shadows of the past. Of course, atheists may acknowledge that certain things are not morally right, but they do not know *why* they are morally wrong; they have no answer to the grand "why" question. Even the non-religious philosopher Jürgen Habermas expressed as his conviction that the ideas of freedom and social co-existence are based on the Jewish notion of justice and the Christian ethics of love. As he puts it, "Up to this very day there is no alternative to it."[19]

For these reasons the writer Fyodor Dostoyevsky was ultimately right when he showed us in his novel *The Brothers Karamazov* that without God all things are permissible; without God's eternal "Beyond," there wouldn't be eternal moral laws and we would be mere animals. Let me make clear that Dostoyevsky is not claiming that without God there would be no moral rules, for even in atheistic societies there are moral rules. What he does claim through the character Ivan is that nothing is *always* wrong because everything is permitted, at least at some point and under some circumstances.[20] Without God, moral absolutism becomes moral relativism. In other words, if God is dead, Ivan himself must take ultimate responsibility for the moral order of the world. He would become the moral commander-in-chief.

Let me take this thought one step farther: Without God we wouldn't even have any moral rights. The United States Declaration of

---

[19] Jürgen Habermas, Ciaran Cronin, and Max Pensky, *Time of Transitions* (Cambridge: Polity Press, 2006), 150-151. See also Eduardo Mendieta, ed., *Religion and Rationality: Essays on Reason, God, and Modernity* (Cambridge, MA: MIT Press, 2002), 149.

[20] R. R. Reno, "Relativism's Moral Mission," *First Things* 222 (2012), 3-5.

Independence sees very clearly that our human rights are God-given rights and that otherwise we wouldn't have any:

> We hold these truths to be self-evident, that all men are created equal, that they are endowed by their Creator with certain unalienable Rights, that among these are Life, Liberty and the pursuit of Happiness.

These are divine birthrights. Without God, we would have no *right* to claim any rights. If rights really came from men, and not God, men could take them away at any time; and they certainly have tried to do so.

However, do not confuse these moral rights with civil rights such as the right to vote at elections or drive a car or hold public office, which are rights attained gradually as the person matures and are actually not rights but entitlements. And do not equate legal laws with moral laws in too easy a fashion. Dr. Martin Luther King Jr. could not have put it better:

> There are just and there are unjust laws.... A just law is a man made code that squares with the moral law or the law of God. An unjust law is a code that is out of harmony with the moral law. To put it in the terms of St. Thomas Aquinas, an unjust law is a human law that is not rooted in eternal and natural law.[21]

So that even if something is legal, it might still be immoral, for what we call legal is not necessarily based on moral values, but rather on moral evaluations. Slavery, for instance, was legally right at one point, and now abortion is, but that doesn't necessarily make them morally right. Laws that subordinate the rights of anyone to those of others are always unjust. Beyond these principles, the relationship between morality and legality is rather intricate. When moral consensus fades—as it did in 1535 in the time of Thomas More and as it does now in our times—society usually turns to law. But when morality is no longer widely shared, the law begins to falter as well, making society and culture teeter on the brink of chaos.

To put it clearly, law cannot be divorced from morality—and, as we found out, morality cannot be divorced from the "Grand Beyond." As

---

[21] In his 1963 *Letter from Birmingham Jail.*

a consequence, law, morality, and religion are strongly intertwined. When religion starts to fade in society, a cascade of effects sets in and starts a dangerous domino effect. As I said earlier, moral values have an added dimension and therefore must be derived from a different realm—from the "Grand Beyond."

Let us wrap up our discussion about rationality and morality: humans are living beings, but unlike other living beings, they are also rational and moral beings. The rational and moral capabilities of human beings are unparalleled in the animate world. Dogs may appear to be "caring" and "dedicated," but they do not feel any moral obligations; and chimpanzees may look "smart," but they are not rational and have no common sense or sound judgment. From this it follows that rationality and morality haven't come down to us from our pre-human ancestors via our umbilical cords.

Rationality and morality do not even seem to be programmed in the DNA of our genes. Had rationality been genetically programmed, we could skip many years of education and would not need rules of logic, math, methodology, and language to help us think more rationally. And had morality been encoded in our genes, we wouldn't need ethical rules for us to behave morally. The Ten Commandments may have been etched in stone, but certainly not in our genes.

Rationality and morality are also alike in their being objective and absolute, which entitles them to claim universal validity. They both defy relativism, whether the relativism is of the intellectual or moral kind. Had they been encoded in our genes, however, they would not have any objective, universal, or absolute validity; and as a consequence, we would never be able to distinguish truth from untruth, or right from wrong.

You might think rationality and morality are something for science to explain, but the situation is actually reversed: they explain and guide science. If we were only the fortuitous effects of physical causes, we would have no other measures of rationality and morality but ourselves. Philosophically, as well as historically, it was on the hotbed of rationality and morality that science was able to emerge and prosper. These keep science alive and upright.

Rational rules as well as moral obligations are just "evident." It is plainly evident that there is order in this world and that like causes produce like effects—there is just no demonstration for it. It is equally evident that it is wrong to kill other human beings; do not ever ask why not, for there is no solid proof. I have nothing to offer as proof that I should do what I should do. So the question is where their "evidence" comes from.

Rationality and morality are gifts of creation, not products of evolution; they are impregnated in our minds and souls by our Maker—a gratuitous gift from our Creator. They are "evident" because they are "God-given"—our "birth-rights," so to speak. Nothing else can explain why we are rational and moral beings. Without God, we have no *reason* to trust our reasoning, and we have no *right* to claim any rights. That is why atheism is an acid that eats away the ground of all rationality and morality. When you take them away, we are back where we came from—animals. Our bodies do come from "below," which is the Earth and the animal world, but our minds come from "above."

So who decides what is true and right? It is certainly not up to us to decide what is true; such a decision depends on the laws of nature in the cosmic design. And it is definitely not up to us to decide what is right, for that depends on the natural law anchored in the cosmic design of creation. Decisions like these are ultimately beyond our control. All we have to do is obediently listen to what the cosmic design—which is the Creator's design—tells us through reason.[22]

We as human beings can make rational and moral decisions. History isn't an accident; history is a choice, for life is a series of choices, from beginning to end. And choices can be rational as well as irrational, moral as well as immoral.

Before we close, let me get some unexpected help from a source far above suspicion—the mathematician Kurt Gödel. He rigorously and mathematically proved in his so-called incompleteness theorem that no coherent system—not even the system of science—can be completely closed; it must contain statements that can be stated but not decided within that system. To prove the consistency of the system requires an "act of faith." In other words, any coherent system

---

[22] Not surprisingly, Isaac Newton had the strong conviction that God could have made the world differently if He wished. That's why particles have certain forces and not others, or planetary orbits have certain parameters and not others. See Isaac Newton, *Opticks*, Query 31.

is essentially incomplete and needs additional "help" from outside the system.[23] Gödel even went so far as to believe that we can't give a credible account of reality itself without invoking God.[24] Or in the words of the famous physicist, Nobel Laureate, and founder of quantum physics, Max Planck:

> Both religion and natural science require a belief in God for their activities; to the former He is the starting point, and to the latter the goal of every thought process.[25]

Science can't possibly explain all of what makes us what we are. Apparently, it is not just a clockwork mechanism that makes us tick; there is so much more to it. Let us catch all of this in a motto: faith and reason!

---

[23] Francesco Berto, *There's Something about Gödel: The Complete Guide to the Incompleteness Theorem.* (Hoboken, NJ: John Wiley and Sons, 2010).

[24] See David Goldman, "The God of the Mathematicians," *First Things*, 205 (2010): 45-50.

[25] Lecture, "Religion and Natural Science" (1937) in Max Planck and Frank Gaynor (trans.), *Scientific Autobiography and Other Papers* (New York: Philosophical Library, 1949), 184.

Intermission 6A

The Boundary Conditions of the Universe

All scientific laws operate within the so-called boundary conditions or restraints. There are a number of physical constants that are known, such as the speed of light and the force of gravity, that are not derivable from any known theory. If the values of these constants were a little different the cosmos as we know it would not be possible. For example, the law of gravitation is constrained within the boundaries set by general relativity for a specific average density of matter; otherwise a cosmological catastrophe would be generated

All other physical factors are causally determined by these more fundamental constants. Is it possible, though, that some of these fundamental constants may in time be derived themselves? For instance, at one time the boiling point of water was taken as a physical constant, but is now considered the result of quantum mechanical laws. In time, the speed-of-light constant may be tied to Planck's constant defining the smallest possible unit of space and time. However, even if all constants were ever to be derived from one single unified theory, we would still be left with the metaphysical question: where does this very theory come from?

No matter what the outcome will be, science will always search for a more complex underlying order at a more fundamental level. This can be seen in what has happened to Kepler's planetary laws when they were derived from Newton's law of gravity, and to Newton's law of gravity when it was deduced from Einstein's law of general relativity. To quote the famous astrophysicist Sir James Jeans again, "the universe begins to look more like a great thought than a great machine."[1] His essential point is that physics is beginning to discover

---

[1] James Jeans, *The Mysterious Universe* (Cambridge University Press, 1930), Chap. 5.

more and more that the universe has an intrinsic rationality, a cosmic order, which governs all that science is trying to decipher.

Yet what the universe and man made machines have in common is the fact that they follow the same rule: they are only useful because the laws of nature have been harnessed within certain boundary conditions or restraints. In man made machines, these restraints attest their design. But why wouldn't the same hold for the "living machines" in nature?

Some people think that this idea of a cosmic design comes close to the so-called anthropic principle. There are many versions of this principle, but it typically asserts that our universe is uniquely "fine-tuned" to give rise to life and even human life. This would entail that the universe must have somehow "known" that we were coming. To paraphrase Descartes, "I think, therefore the world must be this way." It is true, if the boundary conditions of this universe were even slightly different from what they actually are, our universe would probably not exist, and neither would we. Indeed, the odds against a universe like ours appear to be enormous. Yet it seems that worded this way, the principle is actually circular: The universe had to be this way or we would not be here to comment on it! That is rather trivial and begging the question, isn't it? No wonder objections against the anthropic principle have been plenty:

- If our planet had been suitable for another kind of life, it is that kind of life that would have evolved here.

- Another one: The fact that the actual fine-tuning of constants enabled the emergence of life does not entail that life was predestined to emerge.

- And then there is this one: There could be multiple, parallel universes, and ours happens to be a lucky hit.

- And what about this one: Every possible universe that can contain intelligent life will appear "fine-tuned," no matter how it came along.

- One more: It is not the physical environment of this universe that had to get fine-tuned to life, but the other way around—life had to adapt to the physical environment instead, in the same way as the soil did not develop to grow plants, nor did the nose come along to wear glasses.

–   Or finally: The principle is unscientific, since it neither explains nor predicts any physical constants. So it may be one of those unscientific principles that were discarded in the history of science, such as phlogiston and spontaneous generation.

These kinds of objections are rather serious and do weaken the case for the anthropic principle. Frankly, I am not very impressed by this principle—not only because it does have weak points, but most of all because we do not really need it. I think what I have been stressing so far is located at a much deeper philosophical level. The metaphysical questions I have been raising go far beyond the physical data and constants that scientists have come up with. I am more concerned with questions such as "How can electrons do anything whatever, let alone follow laws?" or "How can organisms do anything whatever, let alone survive?" or "How can biological designs be successful, let alone reproduce themselves?" or "How come this universe is comprehensible to the human mind at all?" Even if physics could ever explain why the universe is the way it is, including its physical constants, we would still be left with the metaphysical question as to where the laws come from that explain all that exists.

The answer to these metaphysical questions is not to be found in some kind of anthropocentric principle, but rather in the "architecture" of the universe. The most fundamental question is: why is its cosmic structure this way? Its explanation is not to be found in itself, because the universe is a contingent entity that calls for an ultimate explanation and ground beyond itself—an orderly Creator, a rational Lawgiver, an intelligent Designer, and a moral Lawgiver. I admit that this explanation is not a logical "must," but it is not mere speculation either; it is a strong pointer toward something, or rather someone, transcending the contingency of our universe. How else could we explain that this universe is orderly and intelligible? I realize that the assumption of a Creator or designer does not explain *why* the universe is this way, but it would still be the best explanation of the fact *that* the universe is this way.

Intermission 6B

What Obscures the Grand Beyond

The greatest enemy of metaphysics is ontological reductionism. Reductionism claims that there is nothing more than atoms, molecules, DNA, genes, and neurons behind physics. Reductionists fail to tell model and reality apart. As we found out earlier, science reduces complex entities to a manageable model related to an analyzable problem as a successful way of doing research. But after reducing reality to a simplified model, we should not declare the model to be the new reality. Yet that is exactly what reductionism does; it declares "the real thing" as "nothing but" the simplified model. So reductionists end up saying that an organism is "really nothing but" a collection of genes, that a human being is "really nothing but" a string of DNA or a pack of neurons, that human values are "really nothing but" the outcome of natural selection, that altruism is "really nothing but" hidden self-interest, that thinking is "really nothing but" a series of firings along neurons, that the unborn baby is "really nothing but" a blob of cells, and that a human being is "really nothing but" a mathematical or statistical number. The reductionist explanation is used repeatedly.

Some scientists have tried a different strategy, with the same outcome. They state that physics always has the last word in observation because the observers themselves are physical. But why not then say that psychology always has the last word because these observers make for very interesting psychological objects as well. Either statement is nonsense; observers are neither physical nor psychological or whatever, but they can indeed be studied from a physical, biological, psychological, or statistical viewpoint—which is a different "ball game."

Here is where we must enter metaphysical territory. Reductionism, or what C. S. Lewis called "nothing-buttery," is the fallacy you will frequently hear when scientists leave their own territory; when they leave their own area of expertise and blow it up to immense proportions. Thus they become poor philosophers without schooling in the field of metaphysics. Like some movie stars, some scientists abuse their fame to also broadcast their worldviews—or lack thereof—convinced that their professional or scientific expertise guarantees the quality of any other beliefs they have. The physical chemist Peter Atkins even has the audacity to exclaim that "scientists...are privileged...to see further into the truth than any of their contemporaries."[1] But I would tell him, do not let plumbers advise you on your electrical wiring. Yet we hear such arrogant, overconfident, and all-pervasive statements again and again: according to the DNA co-discoverer Francis Crick, "You're nothing but a pack of neurons"[2]; Marvin Minsky, a pioneer in the field of artificial intelligence, was famous for stating that we are nothing but "machines made of meat"[3]; according to the biologist Richard Dawkins, we are only a cluster of "independent and selfish DNA replicators;"[4] according to the psychiatrist Sigmund Freud, you are only "a bundle of instincts."[5] And the list could go on and on: According to such "gurus," you are nothing but.... Was Archie Bunker right after all in calling his son-in-law "meathead"?

Neglecting what is outside one's scope may be a wise scientific strategy, but denying what lies outside one's horizon goes one step

---

[1] Peter Atkins, "The Limitless Power of Science," *Nature's Imagination: The Frontiers of Scientific Vision*, eds., John Cornwell and Freeman Dyson (Oxford: Oxford University Press, 1995), 121.

[2] Francis Crick, *The Astonishing Hypothesis* (New York: Charles Scribner's Sons, 1994), 1.

[3] Marvin Minsky, *The Emotion Machine: Commonsense Thinking, Artificial Intelligence, and the Future of the Human Mind.* (New York: Simon & Schuster, 2007).

[4] Richard Dawkins, *The Selfish Gene*, Thirtieth Anniversary edition (Oxford: Oxford University Press, 2006), Chap. 12.

[5] "Introductory Lectures on Psychoanalyis" [1916], in James Strachey, ed., *The Standard Edition of the Complete Psychological Works of Sigmund Freud* (London: Hogarth Press, 1963), Vol. 16, 284-285.

farther, actually a step too far, turning science into an unwarranted ideology. It is like stating that highways do not exist because they do not feature on railroad maps. Science can create maps, but it can never claim there are no other maps. Science can never transcend or surpass itself by saying that science is all there is in the universe, for it would be an illegitimate claim made from outside the territory of science. Such claims are called scientism; but scientism is self-defeating, it violates its own rules: If it is true, it makes itself false. How could science itself ever prove that science is the only way of finding truth? That would be like an electric generator running on its own electricity.

Our response to reductionism should be that there is much more to life than science, for as noted in Chapter 1, there is so much that "counts" in life than can be counted. Science just *cannot* account for all that needs to be accounted for. The astonishing successes of science have not been gained by answering every kind of question but precisely by refusing to do so. If human beings were indeed "nothing but" DNA, they would be very fragile creatures; and even this very claim would be worth nothing more than the DNA that supposedly produced that claim. Shackled in physics, we would be stifled. Obviously, we need more than physics—so let us go for metaphysics.

Chapter 7

A New Neuroscience

In the previous chapters, I have argued that it is not molecules, DNA, or not even neurons that make you "tick." This is obviously contrasted with the current paradigm of neuroscience. Here we borrow the Kuhnian term *paradigm* that stands for a collection of rules on how to solve scientific puzzles.[1] The current paradigm of neuroscience—which I will now call the old paradigm—is too materialistic, too deterministic, and too reductionistic to do justice to the unique position of living human beings in the world. The state of neuroscience calls for a new paradigm.

I am not suggesting that all neuroscientists now adhere rigidly to the old paradigm, but a majority obviously do. There is a great deal of resistance to a new paradigm, because the old paradigm has been so successful and a new paradigm, the way I see it, is suffused with metaphysics. And metaphysics has become a "dirty" word in certain circles. Who wants to bring metaphysics into science? Who would want to replace "precise" physical explanations with "vague" metaphysical concepts?

Indeed, we might ask, who would want to do this, especially at a time when the old neuroscience is flourishing more than ever! Why don't we keep working inside, to use Imre Lakatos' term for a scientific strategy, the existing progressive research program.[2] The current programs appear to still have many promising prospects. I can mention one in particular, which following the language of Olaf Sporns, is called the Human Connectome Project. It is comparable in a

---

[1] Since first writing *The Structure of Scientific Revolutions*, Thomas Kuhn conceded in the postscript to the 1970 edition that he used "paradigm" in an ambiguous sense and should have narrowed it to a "disciplinary matrix."

[2] Imre Lakatos (1922–1974) was a Hungarian philosopher of mathematics and science. He is known for his theories that classified research as progressive or degenerate.

way to the very successful Human Genome Project that was in progress a decade ago.[3] In recent times, several research teams have devised ways to make magnetic resonance brain scans seven times faster and analyze neural connections fifty times quicker than a year earlier. Based on these developments, neuroscientists hope and plan to document the basic wiring of the brain. Since the human brain contains about 100 billion neurons linked by more than 100 trillion synapses, researchers are developing ways to automate the mapping of this gigantic network of synapses. They are finding hints that electrical signals are relayed through a series of central "hubs" in the brain. Who would want to stop such a promising paradigm or research program? I certainly do not, but I would also point out that the current neurological approach is missing out on many important vistas. There are so many indications and arguments that the existing paradigm, or research program, is neglecting many essential features of the human mind by reducing mental states to neural states. So we need something more, something better.

To explain the need for something better I will introduce a pyramid as a "visual" representation of the several "levels" of reality. Starting at the bottom of the pyramid with the level of physical causes these levels look like this:

- the level of physical causes

- the level of biological functions

- the level of emotional motives

- the level of intentions

- the level of rational decisions and moral directives

- and finally, the level of grounds and destinations.

This description is not exhaustive, neither is it exclusive. There can be discussion about certain details, but what I am proposing is that we at least acknowledge that there are *levels*. When I say, "I wanted to go, but my legs didn't let me," I am actually jumping between two levels— from the level of intentions ("I myself") back to the level of causes ("my leg problems"). Sometimes such a jump is legitimate but often it

---

[3] In 1995, the Indiana University neuroscientist Olaf Sporns dubbed the nervous system's tangle of neurons and synapses the "connectome."

98

is not. To say, "I didn't want to do this, but my glands made me do it" is only an excuse for dodging my moral responsibilities at the higher level. Similarly, moral responsibility is avoided in the case of claiming that what is "fit" on a biological level is automatically "good" at a moral level; or when advocates of eugenics declare that genetic diversity among humans entitles us to treat those humans differently in a moral sense. They illegally jump from the level of causes or functions to the level of moral values. In particular, consider the evolutionists' claim that we could not come here through God's creation because we came here through evolution; they are confusing the level of grounds with the level of causes.

The pyramid may also help us to more fully and more accurately assess the world around us. For example, what was the driving force behind Hitler's gas chambers? No doubt, the cyanide-based insecticide Zyklon B did the killing—that is at the level of causes. But wasn't there much more to it? Strong emotions of anger and hate, feelings of superiority, were all working together—but at another level. Further, these emotions were propelled and reinforced by elements on yet another level—reasons and decisions coming from a racist worldview. Is that the end of the story? No, there was also Hitler's immorality, his lack of a conscience steered by sound moral values. Where did his immorality come from? Since Hitler had no connection with the level of religiosity, there was nothing to keep his morality in line. Apparently we have many factors occurring here at many different levels—not all tangible, but all equally real.

Our pyramid conveys another important message: science may seem to take our sense of reality down several notches, but do not let that fool you. Science operates at "lower" levels, but it usually ignores the "higher" levels that are beyond its reach that are not measurable and quantifiable. Yet science certainly cannot maintain that those levels do not exist.

Each level in the pyramid adds a new dimension to the level below it, and consequently none of these levels can be reduced wholly to any of the lower levels. Rational decisions, for instance, cannot be fully reduced to factors at lower levels, such as electrical impulses or chemical signals. Neither can moral values be reduced to mere rational considerations or emotional motives, and certainly not to biological functions or physical causes.

The underlying question is essentially as follows: what are the notions basic to our outlook on life? Everyone must accept physical causality as a definite valid perspective; many will also accept functionality in biology as well as emotionality in psychology. All these choices are "matter-of-fact" issues. However, some people, indoctrinated by scientism, would claim that this is as far as they can go, because they consider the scientific method to be the only way of finding truth. They want us to believe that science can account for all that needs to be accounted for; they have the unfounded conviction that the domain of scientific discourse is absolutely limitless. They believe there is no corner of the universe, no dimension of reality, no feature of human existence beyond its reach.

But we must ask these devotees of scientism what causes them to make such a claim. Certainly not science itself we found out. We cannot use science to prove that science is the only way of finding truth, for such a claim can be made only from outside the territory of science. Even if we were to agree that the scientific method gives us more testable results than other sources of knowledge, this would not entitle us to claim that only the scientific method gives us genuine knowledge of reality. This is true even when we admit that in general the power of strict proof grows weaker when the field of reference becomes wider. Logic and mathematics, for example, have a strong power of proof, but those happen to be about very little, their field of reference being narrow. Religion, on the other hand, has the reverse problem: it has a much wider reference but consequently loses some power of proof.

Let me use the following analogy to explain what is so dubious about the claim of scientism: although a web browser is a perfect tool to find any website we want to visit, would this entitle us to state that reality consists only of websites? Of course not! Beside the questions of accuracy or prediction, there is another problem with such a claim. Scientific statements can be true or false, but the things they are about—quarks, atoms, molecules, and cells—are physical or material, and are never true or rational. How could there be truth to what science claims if everything were merely material? Or stated positively, there must be more than what science is focused on. That is why scientism "has not a foot to stand on."

Earlier, in the first chapter, we discussed the problem of self-reference. To apply the self-reference to scientism means this: if scientism claims there is only physical matter, it implies that such a *claim* does not and cannot exist because claims are not physical; and if we think that such a claim does exist, there must be more than physical matter in this universe. When we deny the existence of immaterial things, we also deny the existence of our own immaterial denial. Scientism in fact steps outside scientific territory to claim that there is nothing outside scientific territory. It declares that everything outside science is a despicable form of metaphysics, without realizing that anyone who rejects metaphysics can do so only on *metaphysical* grounds.

So if scientism is an illegitimate claim, what then makes some believe that causality as it occurs on lower levels in the pyramid is more "real" than rationality and morality at higher levels? True, the domain of causality is about what is tangible, measurable, countable, and quantifiable. But I would ask again if winking is less "real" than blinking. A camera may not be able to catch the difference, but we all know there is a difference; there is something behind a wink that a camera cannot capture. Who could or would deny such an obvious fact? If you do, you must have been brainwashed to accept that what instruments cannot capture can not and does not exist.

Due to scientific developments, our cosmos has been significantly expanded in regard to what can be touched, measured, or counted. But be aware, what is called the "scientific world" is just one aspect of the "real world." The fact that other aspects are beyond the scope of science doesn't make them less "real" or less "factual" or less "objective" or less "valid." You cannot just choose what to neglect. Reality is like a jewel with many facets that can be looked at from various angles, with different eyes, but do not claim that you need only look at it from one angle, or from one specific level in the pyramid. There are many more perspectives than what science tries to cover with its barometers, thermometers, and spectrometers. Just as the "physical eye" sees colors in nature, so the "moral eye" sees moral values in life. All these "eyes" are in search of reality, but each one "sees" a different aspect of it.

Finally, there is one more argument: causality is a notion of the human mind and therefore is, in and of itself, based on...well, rationality! So rationality must have a source outside our sensorial experiences—and that source can only be God, as I argued in the previous chapter. If our rationality is "real," it must come from a reality outside our sensorial experiences and must have a cause outside our sensorial experiences. If there is such a thing as real rationality, then only God can be its source.

Yet radical skeptics, followers of David Hume, doubt whether any of the above fundamental levels in the pyramid can be trusted; they deny the validity of almost all aspects of knowledge because we are not supposed to know any truth with certainty. But, you may ask, aren't all scientists supposed to be skeptics? No, they do need a critical mind, but not a skeptical mind. A skeptic finds a flaw in every truth claimed. As a consequence, skepticism makes for a very restrained view of the world—actually so restrained that absolute skeptics cannot even know whether they have a mind to doubt with. Skeptics turn things the wrong way. We often do need to eliminate errors to get to the truth; yet our ultimate goal is not to avoid errors, but to gain truth. We certainly want to *know* rather than to know what we do *not* know. Skeptics, on the other hand, make it their final goal to avoid errors, in denial of the fact that eliminating errors is only a means to gaining truth—so they end up with an all-pervasive mistrust.

All we have discussed so far sounds like old-fashioned metaphysics, and no scientist wants that kind of "jumble," as some call it, to become part of a new paradigm in neuroscience. The high priests of the old paradigm want no "outdated" metaphysical terminology but only "modern" physical explanations. But before we throw metaphysics away, let us examine first how the Hungarian-British physical-chemist and philosopher Michael Polanyi would deal with the separate levels we distinguished in our pyramid.[4] He became famous—some would say infamous—for stating that a machine based on the laws of physics is not explicable by the laws of physics alone, because the structure of a machine is what he calls a "boundary condition" extraneous to the process it delineates.[5] His argument relies on the assumption that boundary conditions supply degrees of freedom that, instead of being random, are determined by higher-level realities whose properties are dependent on, yet distinct from, the lower level from which they emerge.

---

[4] Michael Polanyi, "Life's Irreducible Structure," *Science* 160 (June 1968): 1308–1312.

[5] Polanyi, *The Tacit Dimension* (New York: Doubleday, 1966), 38.

In the case of machines, these boundary conditions were created by the designing mind of its engineer in order to harness the processes regulated by physical laws, but they are irreducible to those laws. It seems to me that this idea has quite some repercussions for the debate on artificial intelligence. All forms of artificial intelligence presume a designing mind, or at least some form of artificial shaping, that creates the right boundary conditions. All machines function according to some human design of constraints, so they are not only based on the laws of physics. We will not pursue the question of artificial intelligence or the so-called technological singularity here.[6]

But how can we apply these thoughts about machines to living entities? Instead of using the pyramid, I will introduce another "visual" tool: the hierarchical structure of living beings. A simplified hierarchy of an organism would look like this:

- an organism

- organs

- cells

- molecules

- particles, and so on.

Each level in the hierarchy is composed of building blocks from "lower" levels, but in itself is also "building material" for "higher" levels. The relation between levels is a part-whole relationship.

What is noteworthy about these hierarchical levels is that each level has properties not shown at lower levels. This phenomenon is called emergence.[7] The properties of water molecules, for instance, do not show up at the level of its components, the hydrogen and oxygen atoms. This same emergence holds for functions such as ventilation, respiration, and oxidation: Ventilation occurs at the level of organisms, respiration at the level of cells, and oxidation at the level of molecules. Polanyi teaches us that principles and processes at a

---

[6] "Technological singularity" refers to a hypothetical greater-than-human intelligence emerging through computers.

[7] See, for instance, James Marcum and G.M.N. Verschuuren, "Hemostatic Regulation and Whitehead's Philosophy of Organism,"*Acta Biotheoretica*, 35 (1986): 123–133.

higher level cannot be derived from principles and processes at a lower level alone, just as it is impossible to derive a grammar from a vocabulary, or a vocabulary from phonetics. Am I advocating here that those new properties "emerge" from nowhere—as if they came "out of nothing"? No I certainly am not, because the relationships between components at a lower level are also a "given" part of the cosmic design. It is those relationships that determine which new properties can emerge at a higher level.

Let us go back once more to the discussion we had in Chapter 2 about the role of DNA. The properties of a cell are of a "higher" level than the properties of a molecule such as DNA, and cannot be derived from the DNA structure alone; DNA does not produce a cell on its own. In turn, the properties of DNA are of a "higher" level than those of its composing atoms; the DNA sequence cannot be derived from physical and chemical laws alone, because it has one specific, particular arrangement out of many possible arrangements that are equivalent in an energetical and physico-chemical sense.[8]

When we apply these insights to our discussion about neuroscience, we should ask neuroscientists at what level they want to work. Is it the level of molecules, especially neurotransmitters, or the level of cells, in particular neurons, or the level of organs, such as the brain, or rather at the level of organisms? The level of organisms would call for mental concepts as well. In the new paradigm for neuroscience that I suggest, I would prefer to focus on the level of entire organisms, and not just their component parts. The mind transcends the brain to the same degree by which life transcends everyday chemistry and physics. The mind is of a "higher level" than the brain, in the same way that the brain is of a "higher level" than its components.

We discussed extensively in the previous chapters how the assumption that the mind is identical to the brain is philosophically— or metaphysically if you wish—incorrect. So the question is this: Should neuroscience explain the mind in terms of the brain, or instead the brain in terms of the mind?

---

[8] I am not going into the discussion here of how specific DNA sequences came along. An account of how a system works is different from how it came into existence.

What are explanations? What does it mean when we explain something? An explanation is a statement that confers intelligibility on a certain phenomenon. That which is to be explained must be explained in terms of things that do not need to be explained. In other words, explanations need "a bedrock" to rest upon. As Ludwig Wittgenstein reminds us, "Explanations come to an end somewhere."[9] The question is which are the things that need not be explained. For most neuroscientists, those things should be located at lower levels of the hierarchy: atoms, molecules, or cells. But why couldn't we look at higher levels? What makes some people believe that the working of DNA is explained better by finding an explanation at a lower level, say in its molecular structure, than by finding an explanation at a higher level in the surrounding cellular structure? Something similar applies to our discussion about neuroscience. The "old" paradigm extends exclusively for lower levels, whereas my new paradigm would preferably start at a higher level. There is no compelling reason why explanations should always go in one direction, macro-to-micro or micro-to-macro. No level has a monopoly, although the old paradigm suggests that is so.

I have made the compelling case that there is indeed such a higher level—the level of mental activities. There is no reason why we cannot use what are called metaphysical concepts such as consciousness, free will, self-reflection, self-determination, self-expression, self-transcendence, self-examination, self-discipline, introspection, and morality as the ground of our explanations. Such concepts are off-limits only for "narrow-minded" scientists who accept only the existence of lower levels. One of these is biologist George Simpson, who is representative of some of his colleagues when he considers human beings purely as biological organisms. This makes him exclaim, "Metaphysics, art, and literature can contribute nothing."[10] The inconsistency and irony of such a stance is that this rejection of metaphysics is based on a *metaphysical* viewpoint regarding what "reality" is supposed to be. Denying the existence of mental activities is in itself a mental activity, and thus leads to contradiction.

---

[9] Ludwig Wittgenstein, *Philosophical Investigations* (New York: Blackwell Publishing, 1953/2001), §1.

[10] George Gaylord Simpson, *Biology and Man* (New York: Harcourt, Brace & World, 1969), 80.

Let me introduce a simple example to clarify the impact of metaphysics on neuroscience. We are told that sixteen million Americans suffer from depression, and now chemical tests are being developed to diagnose this disease. The general assumption behind these tests is clear: if the test is positive, we will have detected something chemical, or at least material, that causes depression and needs adjustment. Indeed, many researchers believe depression is caused by chemical changes in the brain. My objection to this assumption is that nothing forces us to explain any association between depression and a chemical substrate in terms of *causality*. On the other hand, metaphysics can help us search for a "higher" level of mental factors—such as anger, frustration, low self-esteem, separation, rejection, abuse, failure, grief, guilt, lack of faith, or even sinfulness. Instead of using anti-depressants, we should look for the real causes behind them—let us lump them together as "negative thoughts." Perhaps these mental factors are the actual cause of chemical changes, instead of the other way around.

I assume from now on that you agree that human beings do have mental states, distinct from neural states. Can I prove this? No, there is no conceivable observation or deductive argument that will constitute a proof of the existence of consciousness in anything other than oneself. Consciousness is not a diagnostic property. But I think I have adduced enough support for the validity of my metaphysical claims. To reiterate just one argument: without the assumption of a rational mind, the entire structure of the scientific enterprise would collapse. So let us find out what the new paradigm for neuroscience would, could, or should look like.

Intermission 7A

Thinking Animals

The word "Man" comes to us from the archaic Indo-Aryan language Sanskrit. In Sanskrit "Manu," meaning thinking or wise, refers to the essence of human beings, as indeed humans are born to be philosophers. Philosophy may seem a sophisticated endeavor to many; but we note with Aristotle, who in the first sentence of his Metaphysics says "All men by nature desire to know," that each one of us is destined to philosophize at some point in life.[1] No wonder we are called thinking animals.

Because we are "thinking animals," not only *can* we use our minds for philosophical ponderings, but we have *an obligation* in the sense discussed in Chapter 5 to do so; to do anything less would be to reject the gift of reason. As the philosopher Immanuel Kant put it:

> Man is distinguished above all animals by his self-consciousness, by which he is a *"rational animal"* (emphasis added)[2]

However, to acknowledge humans are "thinking animals" might be taken in two ways. On the one hand, placing the emphasis on "thinking" implies that what distinguishes us from other animals is our capacity for thinking—that is, what makes us unique. On the other hand, the designation "animals" might suggest that we came forth from the animal world—so that our rational thinking must have roots in the animal world, thus diminishing our uniqueness.

---

[1] Aristotle, (1.980a21).

[2] Immanuel Kant, *Critique of Pure Reason*, Preface and 8: 414 (cf. *Lectures on Anthropology*, 7: 321, where he speaks of "an animal endowed with the capacity of reason," but not yet "a rational animal").
In the *Nicomachean Ethics* I.13, Aristotle had already stated that the human being has a rational principle, which view became very common in Scholastical philosophy.

Evolutionists will take the latter interpretation, quoting Darwin's famous admonition—that the difference between animals and man is one of degree, not of kind. In line with this doctrine, humans ought to be degraded to glorified animals, and/or animals ought to be inflated to pre-humans, humans-in-the-making so to speak. There have been experiments made to demonstrate this point. Let us examine the following classical experiment as a test case.[3] Rats were trained to expect food to drop into a little tray after a certain sound. Next those rats went through a second training in which they found food in the tray without a sound, but with a vomative in it. After these two training sessions, we might expect that a sound would make them go to the tray (as a result of the first training), but then they would not eat the food (as a result of the second training). In practice, they gradually stopped going to the tray!

The scientists who did this experiment adopted the explanation of conditional reasoning. They claimed the rats had two expectations and from these made a logical inference based on a mental concept. Supposedly for the rats:

1. "sound causes food" (if A then B), and

2. "food causes vomiting" (if B then C) —and from this, these smart rats deduced the following thought:

3. "sound causes vomiting" (if A then C).

In other words, "food" (B) had become a mental concept, so it acted as a logical link between a sound and vomiting, making vomiting a reason to stop going to the tray. So are those rats logical thinkers endowed with phenomenal minds?

This experiment, as well as many others, that claim to demonstrate reasoning in animals has a problem: The test results taken as evidence for conditional reasoning can equally well be explained by associative conditioning (A and B, or B and C). Hence, opting for the assumption of logical reasoning is arbitrary if we do not have additional compelling evidence. The rats learned to associate sound with food (A and B) and food with vomiting (B and C), so they

---

[3] Holland, P. C., Rescorla, R. A., "Second-order conditioning with food unconditioned stimulus," *Journal of Comparative and Physiological Psychology*, 88 (1975): 459-467.

did not touch the food in step 2, hence were not rewarded, and thus gradually stopped going to the tray. Depending on the paradigm one works in, humans are unique or humans are glorified animals, either explanation is compelling. But if you do accept conditional reasoning, which has much wider ramifications, you would need additional arguments that are not presented. So, in fact, the reason why one would select reasoning over conditioning would be ideological—evolutionism that is!

In order to prove their case, the experimenters also trained a control group. These rats went through the same first training ("sound causes food"), but the second training was modified: Instead of finding food with a vomative in it, they received only a vomitive and no food. If these rats were to become "frustrated" by continually going to a tray without food, they would stop going to the tray. In practice, however, this group kept going after each sound, although there was no food in the tray! From this, the researchers concluded that these rats did not get tired of going for nothing but must have had a "logical reason" to keep going.

Again I question the refusal of these researchers to accept the alternative option—associative conditioning. Like the first group of rats, the second group learned to make the same first association, "sound with food" (A and B), but the second association was "no-food with vomiting" (not-B and C), so they kept going to the tray for absent food—which, by the way, does not demonstrate rationality or logic. If in fact these rats were "great thinkers," they surely wouldn't act that way.

But, as noted earlier, there is a difference between animal intelligence and human rationality. Intelligence can, indeed, provide helpful survival tools, but it is our rationality that allows us to understand and explain the world we live in. Ultimately we can agree with Immanuel Kant that humans are the only animals who are rational and characterized by the use of mental concepts and moral reasoning.

Interestingly, it was an evolutionary biologist, the British-born geneticist and noted neo-Darwinian thinker, J. B. S. Haldane, who heralded the power of reasoning when he made the following statement:

If my mental processes are determined wholly by the motions of atoms in my brain, I have no reason to suppose that my beliefs are true...and hence I have no reason for supposing my brain to be composed of atoms.[4]

---

[4] J. B. S. Haldane, *Possible Worlds and Other Essays* (Harper and Brothers, 1928), 209.

Intermission 7B

Do Machines Think Like We Do?

The debate on artificial intelligence (AI) centers around the following question: Would an appropriately programmed computer with the right inputs and outputs *simulate* a mind or actually *have* a mind? The first version is uncontroversial. But the second version, called strong AI, would have enormous repercussions if it were true. Certainly it could upset the arguments concerning mental, immaterial minds that I am using in this book. So let us look more closely into strong AI.

The declarations of the first wave of AI researchers reflected strong AI. For example, in 1955 AI founder, Herbert Simon declared that:

> there are now in the world machines that think, that learn and create...[We can explain] how a system composed of matter can have the properties of mind.[1]

John Haugeland, an influential voice in cognitive science, wrote in 1983 that "we are, at root, computers ourselves."[2] Specifically, strong AI represents the view that suitably programmed computers can understand natural language and have other mental capabilities similar to the humans whose abilities they mimic in playing chess or using language.

From the last decades of the twentieth century the arguments between those who were opposed to the concept that machines can think and the strong AI visionaries of technology were hotly debated. In January 1990, the popular monthly *Scientific American* took the

---

[1] Quoted in Russell, Stuart J., and Norvig, Peter, *Artificial Intelligence: A Modern Approach* (2nd ed.), (Upper Saddle River, NJ: Prentice Hall, 2003), 21, 17.

[2] Haugeland, John (1985), *Artificial Intelligence: The Very Idea*, (Cambridge, MA: MIT Press. 1985), 2.

debate to a general scientific audience. One of the main attacks against strong AI assertions comes from the Berkeley philosopher John Searle.[3] He introduced what is widely known now as the "Chinese Room Argument"—first presented in 1983.[4]

Searle's Chinese Room argument can be summarized as follows:

> Imagine a native English speaker who knows no Chinese locked in a room full of boxes of Chinese symbols (a data base) together with a book of instructions for manipulating the symbols (the program). Imagine that people outside the room send in other Chinese symbols which, unknown to the person in the room, are questions in Chinese (the input). And imagine that by following the instructions in the program the man in the room is able to pass out Chinese symbols which are correct answers to the questions (the output). The program enables the person in the room to pass the Turing Test for understanding Chinese but he does not understand a word of Chinese.[5]

The question Searle poses is: does the machine understand Chinese? Or is it merely simulating the ability to understand Chinese? If you can carry on an intelligent conversation with an unknown partner, does this imply that your statements are *understood*? Strong AI claims that the ability to converse shows understanding; while in contrast Searle argues that we cannot describe what the machine is doing as "thinking." Since it does not think, it does not have a "mind" in anything like the normal sense of the word. Therefore, he concludes, strong AI is mistaken.

What Searle denotes by "understanding" is what philosophers call intentionality. Intentionality is the property of being *about* something, of having *content*. In the nineteenth century, psychologist Franz Brentano reintroduced this term from scholastic philosophy

---

[3] See his *Intentionality: An Essay on the Philosophy of Mind*, (Cambridge: Cambridge University Press, 1983) and his *The Rediscovery of Mind*, (Cambridge, MA: The MIT Press, 1992).

[4] Searle, John, "Minds, Brains and Programs," *Behavioral and Brain Sciences*, 3 (1983): 417–457.

[5] "The Chinese Room," in R.A. Wilson and F. Keil (eds.), *The MIT Encyclopedia of the Cognitive Sciences*, (Cambridge, MA: MIT Press, 1999).

and held that intentionality was the "mark of the mental."[6] The term was also widely used by the philosopher Edmund Husserl. Then Gottlob Frege made it a standard practice in analytic philosophy to investigate the intentional structure of human thought by inquiring into the logical structure of the language used by speakers to express it or to ascribe it to others.[7] In other words, beliefs are intentional states—meaning they have propositional content, such as "one believes that in this case the given proposition is true."

Needless to say, Searle's argument has been attacked from many sides. I won't go into those discussions here. However, Searle's thought experiment appeals to our strong intuition that what the theoretical computer in the "Chinese Room" accomplishes, does not amount to understanding Chinese. The consensus now appears to be that Searle is quite right on this point—no matter how you program a computer; it will not be a mind and will not understand natural language. This has not constituted a final defeat for strong AI which appears to live on in the pursuit of the "singularity"—defined as the point where nonbiological intelligence will match and exceed the range and subtlety of human intelligence. But I have not seen a defeat of the Chinese Room argument.

---

[6] Brentano's *Irreducibility Thesis* claims that intentionality is an irreducible feature of mental phenomena, and since no physical phenomena could exhibit it, mental phenomena could not be a species of physical phenomena.

[7] Frege described the following puzzle (1892): How can one rationally hold two distinct singular beliefs that are both about one and the same object?

Chapter 8

The Shadow of a Paradigm Shift

The first issue to be considered is what kind of concepts is permitted in the new paradigm, for this determines which kinds of hypotheses are acceptable in the new neuroscience. The physicist and philosopher of science Karl Popper used to tease his audience by shouting, "Observe!"—which necessarily evokes the question "Observe what?"[1] There is no observation without some form of expectation. The problem we have here, I believe, is best expressed by the good old philosopher Plato, although in a slightly different context: "How would you search for what is unknown to you?" Plato noticed a seeming paradox here: we are in search of something "unknown"—otherwise we wouldn't need to search any more. And yet it must be "known" at the same time—otherwise we wouldn't know what to search for, or wouldn't even know if we had found what we were searching for.[2] That is the reason why we need concepts, which are usually couched as hypotheses. These concepts work like "searchlights" that can help us illuminate what was in "darkness" before.[3]

---

[1] Karl R. Popper, *Conjectures and Refutations: The Growth of Scientific Knowledge* (London: Routledge Classics, 1963/2002), 61.

[2] Meno (80d). It is in an ethical context that Plato poses this question to Socrates: "How would you search for what is unknown to you? For, what idea would you have of what you are looking for, while it is unknown to you? Even if you would come across it, how could you know that it is the same as what you did not know?" This is used as a key passage in Th. Kisiel, "Zu einer Hermeneutik naturwissenschaftlicher Entdeckung," *Zeitschrift für allgemeine Wissenschaftliche Theorie*, 2 (1971): 203.

[3] The term "searchlight" is borrowed from and explained in Karl R. Popper, *Objective Knowledge*, revised edition (Oxford: Clarendon Press, 1979), Appendix 1: "The Bucket and the Searchlight—Two Theories of Knowledge."
As early as 1865, Claude Bernard called a theory a "light" instead of an

In observation, one is both a passive "spectator" and an active "creator" at the same time. We do not "have" observations like we have sensorial experiences—we "make" observations.[4] If scientists were mere passive observers, cameras would certainly qualify as the best scientists! Philosophical giants such as Aristotle and Thomas Aquinas would put it this way: all we know about the world comes through our senses, but this is then processed by the intellect that extracts from sensory experiences that which is intelligible.

That is where the need for concepts comes in. Concepts are the main building blocks of both our thoughts and our statements. They are the result of abstraction. When we see a red flower, we form the abstraction of redness, phrased in the concept "redness." We never see redness itself or on its own, but only things that can be red. In the real world, there is no redness; it is an abstraction. Abstraction allows us to find similarities in the midst of dissimilarities. Even when we call something "unique," we classify and categorize it with other "unique" things that are similar in being "unique" but dissimilar in everything else.

However, similarity is not visible until we know already what it is that "similar" cases have in common. We need to identify first what is relevant to our problem, because similarity cannot be established until it has been identified in a word, or actually in a concept. We cannot mechanically infer from a few cases to all similar cases until their similarity has been conceptualized first. Since things can be "alike" in many ways, we need a unifying concept of similarity first in order to classify and categorize things. Before we can "notice" a carnivore, we need the "notion" of a carnivore first.

In other words, there is no re-cognition without cognition. Therefore, scientists are in need of imaginative, bold ideas as outlined in what is called a hypothesis; it is this very hypothesis that makes them "see" the similarity that they couldn't see before. Alas, hypotheses and theories do not spontaneously emerge from observation. Biologists, for instance, couldn't see the similarity in

---

absolute authority: Bernard, *An Introduction to the Study of Experimental Medicine* (New York, Dover Publications, 1957, trans.), 40.

[4] Karl R. Popper, *Objective Knowledge*, revised edition (Oxford: Clarendon Press, 1979), 342.

building blocks between animals and plants until the concept of a cell had been established; neither could they see the similarity between leprosy and tuberculosis until the concept of bacteria had become available. Seeing similarities has been the main driving force behind science. Seeing the similarity between falling apples and revolving planets gave Newton the concept of gravity. Seeing a similarity between the wing of a bird and the hoof of a horse gave Darwin the concept of adaptation.

In the new paradigm of neuroscience, we should be able to discern similarities that the old paradigm, by definition, could not discern or even tolerate—more specifically, similarities in *mental* phenomena. No matter whether some people denigrate them as being "metaphysical" concoctions, they can be powerful "searchlights" in the new paradigm of neuroscientific research.

A notable feature of the new paradigm is that metaphysical concepts may open up unexpected research areas that the old paradigm would ignore. There is one specific metaphysical concept in particular that couldn't feature in the old paradigm—evil. How would the new paradigm fare with such an issue? It seems rather obvious that people with perfectly normal brains do evil things all the time. The question is, for instance, what is going on in the brain when the mind is considering evil actions?

For scientists of the old paradigm, evil belongs to a superseded and superstitious world of "black and white." They think we do not do anything wrong, but things just go wrong—due to our genes, hormones, and what have you. They consider evil to be some kind of disease located somewhere in a gene, a gland, a temporal lobe, or some such physical object.

However, we know intuitively that evil is an ontological, metaphysical reality, something to watch out for. What do I mean by this? First of all, I note that evil is not a "thing"—like a dark cloud or a dangerous storm or a faulty gene. St. Augustine puts it this way: evil exists only in the sense that it subtracts from the good. Thomas Aquinas further elaborates on this issue. In one of his last books, *De Malo*, he says: no being (*essentia*) is evil in itself, for evil is not a thing (*ens* or *res*), not even a reality (*realitas*).[5] So the evil of murder, for

---

[5] Thomas Aquinas, *De Malo*, q. 1, art. 1.

instance, is not a thing—just as an amputation of a limb is not a thing, but rather a lack of something: something "that subtracts from the good." Aquinas often compares this with blindness: Being blind is not some-thing, but whoever happens to be blind is something real; evil is not some-thing on its own, but it can be seen in relation to some-thing good. Or take amputation again: it's not a thing, but lack thereof. Does this mean that evil is not real? Certainly not! As to blindness, the blind person is real, a reality, whereas blindness itself is not a positive some-thing but a lack of eyesight. Evil is real just like an amputation is real, without being a thing. In that specific sense, evil is an ontological, metaphysical reality—as real as blindness and amputation.

We cannot deny the reality of evil. We even have an intuitive assessment of it—as the dictum in the United States Supreme Court on pornography put it, "I know it when I see it."[6] That is not a very precise criterion, but still very effective. "Everyone" knows it is evil when they see the actions of people such as Hitler, Stalin, and Mao. We see how the power of evil enabled these men to spellbind and enslave the minds and spirits of millions, creating a hell ahead of time, right here on Earth. They felt spiritually empowered from "on high"—or from a higher level, if you will. We all know how their intentions, thoughts, beliefs, and their bigoted reasoning shaped human history. Were those mental processes less real than their concentration camps? Somehow, evil is a very serious metaphysical and spiritual "force" in a physical body. Should neuroscience neglect, or even deny, such realities because they are supposedly "metaphysical"? I do not think so.

However, we have to be aware of the following problem: Mental activities may very well qualify to be called "evil," but neural activities cannot. There are evil thoughts, but there are no evil functional magnetic resonance imagings (fMRIs).[7] We cannot take people with "evil" fMRIs off the street, for such would be neuroscientific totalitarianism. It is not their fMRI that is evil, but their mental decisions and ideas. Besides, neural activities found in an

---

[6] Associate Justice Potter Stewart *Jacobellis v. Ohio* (1964).

[7] Functional magnetic resonance imaging (fMRI) is an MRI procedure that measures brain activity by detecting associated changes in blood flow.

fMRI are not a sufficient condition for mental activities, not even evil ones.

A disturbing facet of the old paradigm is the fact that some neuroscientists, declaring neuroscience competent to interrogate morality, believe that neuroscience can show us whether our moral judgments are reliable or not. The problem with this assertion is that the old paradigm doesn't acknowledge morality, so how could it ever scientifically test morality? That is "bootstrap" magic! Science assumes rationality and morality, so it cannot study its own presuppositions. Besides, rationality and morality reside on a level above the phenomena that science studies, so rational and moral principles cannot be derived from principles at a lower level where rationality and morality do not occur. Propositions containing terms that apply to morality cannot be deduced from propositions in which those terms are missing. Of course, these scientists declare morality a biological issue, a matter of genes and natural selection. But it is hardly possible to validate such a claim, as we found out in chapter 5.

Another characteristic of the new paradigm is that neural activity is not—like in the old paradigm—considered a *sufficient* condition for mental activity. Because "metaphysical" concepts must also be considered "emergent," we have to deal with the fact that each hierarchical level has properties not shown at lower levels. As a consequence, principles and processes at the mind level cannot be derived from principles and processes at the brain level, at least not exclusively. In the new paradigm, we should focus on the level of entire organisms and not just their composing parts. The mind transcends the brain to the same degree that life transcends chemistry and physics. The mind is of a "higher level" than the brain, in the same way that the brain is of a "higher level" than its components.

From the fact that the mind transcends the brain follows an important caveat: Even if we discover that certain mental phenomena are associated with certain neural phenomena, this does not entail that these mental phenomena were caused by neural phenomena. Correlation doesn't automatically equal causation. When regions light up on an fMRI, that doesn't explain whether this lit-up state indicates they are causing a certain mental state or just reflecting it. It could very well be, as we discussed before, that the brain is just a material carrier for the mind's immaterial thoughts.

Therefore, the new paradigm needs to find out whether certain mental phenomena always correlate with certain neural phenomena; and furthermore, if they are proportional to the intensity of the mental phenomena. If that is not the case—and mounting evidence indicates it is not—then an important assumption of the old paradigm has actually been falsified. Pain, as noted earlier, can be induced physically, but there is no evidence that this is possible for thoughts too. On the other hand, if we were to find that experimental stimulation of specific neuronal areas would produce a specific mental state or a specific thought, this would be a falsification of an essential component of the new paradigm.

In this regard it should be noted that unlike thoughts, which are of a mental nature, feelings and emotions are physical and biological phenomena that can be physically induced by stimulation of certain brain areas (even animals have those). This is also true of memories stored in the brain, including memories of thoughts once produced by the mind, because memories can be physically stored, similar to the way thoughts can be "stored" on paper. Thoughts can be physically stored in memory, but they cannot be produced in a physical manner.

The new paradigm I propose has another important assumption: the mind may be able to mold the brain, instead of the other way around. It accepts the idea that the mind is at a "higher level" and can thus be in charge of the brain. There is evidence that the neuronal network can carry out instructions given by the mind, and the new paradigm would open the door for more research in this area. The mind may mold the brain like a programmer programs a computer.

By creating new neuronal connections, the mind seems to be able to install new "programs" in the brain. Through goal-setting, self-talk (affirmations), self-examination (evaluations), and mental imagery (visualization), the mind can create new connections in the brain. In fact, there is much more empirical testing needed in this respect. But the new paradigm at least allows for mental training of the brain, similar to what physical training does for the body. Some might call this idea "mind over matter."

Even if scientists from the old paradigm argue that genes affect hormones, and that hormones affect the brain, and that the brain affects our behavior, then the new paradigm would point out that this behavior, in turn, affects the brain again. A similar phenomenon is well known from sports. For instance, strong muscles benefit those who play sports, but in turn, playing sports greatly benefits the development of the muscles. The new paradigm acknowledges that this would also be possible for the brain.

A very salient feature of the new paradigm is the assumption that neural activity not only fails to be a sufficient condition for mental activity, but it may not even be a *necessary* condition. Put differently, mental activity doesn't always correlate with neural activity; in fact, there may be mental activity with hardly any neural activity. This is where the new paradigm opens up new paths to pursue in neuroscience by allowing for the fact that mental activity does not always need neural activity. The mind—that "spooky" metaphysical concept according to the old paradigm—could very well be a powerful metaphysical force in a physical body.

The need for such an assumption becomes even stronger when we consider situations where the most intense subjective experiences correlate with a dampening—or even cessation—of brain activity. In particular, there can be high mental activity without a corresponding high neural activity. What comes to mind are cases of near-death experiences (NDEs) or out-of-body experiences (OBEs) induced by G-LOC,[8] cortical deactivation through the use of high-power magnetic fields, mystical experiences induced through hyper-ventilation, and brain damage caused by surgery or strokes.

I will mention one case study that seems to fit into this new paradigm. The cardiologist Pim van Lommel studied with his team a group of Dutch patients who had been brain-dead from cardiac arrest but were successfully revived. He found that sixty-two patients, eighteen percent, had an NDE while having a flat EEG.[9] There have been many similar observations. What such experiences suggest is that the mind or soul can survive brain-death. If this is confirmed, there could be mind activities without neural activities associated with flat EEGs.

---

[8] G-LOC or G-force-induced loss of consciousness is a term generally used in aerospace physiology to describe a loss of consciousness occurring from excessive and sustained g-forces draining blood away from the brain, causing cerebral hypoxia.

[9] Pim van Lommel, a.o. "Near-death-experience in survivors of cardiac arrest," *The Lancet*, 358 (2001): 2039–2045.

Findings like these can have an enormous impact on the way we think about people who lie in a coma, who have Alzheimer's disease, or who show seriously disabled brain capacity. The fact that they have none or hardly any neural activity doesn't mean that their mental activity has come to a halt as well. Defects in the physical network of neurons or neurotransmitters can prevent the mind from working through bodily activities in the way it had previously, or usually, done. Despite the defects, there can still be something mental that makes them "tick."

Another area of research in keeping with the new paradigm will surely be placebos. A placebo is a "dummy" medication—an inert *inactive* substance, such as sugar, that is thought to have no effect on the condition being treated, and is given to patients to deceive them into thinking that they are receiving a substance that might effect an improvement or cure. Placebos are used in clinical medicine as well as laboratory research to test the effectiveness of a new medication. Because there is a consensus among the medical and scientific establishment that "real" pain or "real" symptoms could respond only to an *active* chemical agent, the reasoning is that a chemical agent can only be proven to be effective if it "beats" an inactive agent in causing actual changes to pain or disease.

Nevertheless, it is clear that placebos are not really without effect. They do have an effect that is called the placebo effect. A placebo intervention may cause patients to *believe* the treatment will change their condition; and this belief can produce a subjective perception of a therapeutic effect, causing the patients to feel their condition has improved. Under the old paradigm, this outcome is essentially an anomaly; placebo effects are a nuisance, something that shouldn't be. Imre Lakatos[10] would consider them part of the "*negative* heuristics" of a research program instructing us which paths of research to *avoid*. A possible solution in line with the old paradigm would be to call the placebo biologically inactive but perhaps psychologically active. If a placebo stops an illness, it must be that either the illness was "all in the mind" and/or that the healing of the illness is "all in the mind." We are led to believe that the illness wasn't real, or the healing wasn't real but was only perceived that way.

---

[10] Imre Lakatos, *The Methodology of Scientific Research Programmes: Philosophical Papers, Volume 1* (Cambridge: Cambridge University Press, 1978).

However, in some medical studies there are patients who are healed by means not explainable scientifically. Sometimes doctors can explain away these results as insignificant or caused by a slight miscalculation in statistics. When this is not possible, doctors describe it as the placebo effect. The fact is that the placebo effect stubbornly remains, no matter how small the number of patients, so it cannot be denied that placebos do have a "real effect."

There is a wide variety of things that exhibit a placebo effect: pharmacological substances, medical devices, sham surgery, sham electrodes implanted in the brain, sham acupuncture, have all exhibited placebo effects. Actually, the common practice of prescribing antibiotics for anything non-bacterial such as a viral cold and the flu can be seen as an example of placebo use. Perhaps homeopathic medicines also belong to this category. So we should question whether the placebo effect is only a "perceived" effect and whether the effect is not only "in the mind" but also in the body.

The basic mechanisms of placebo effects have been investigated since 1978, when it was found that the opioid antagonist naloxone could block placebo painkillers, suggesting that endogenous opioids are involved.[11] A placebo described as a muscle relaxant will cause muscle relaxation and, if described as the opposite, muscle tension.[12] A placebo presented as a stimulant will have this effect on heart rhythm and blood pressure, but, when administered as a depressant, the opposite effect.[13] Also, the entire field of psycho-neuro-immunology is based on the notion that psychological factors cause physiological changes in our body's immune system which are measurable and quantifiable, showing that placebos produce physical changes in diseases rather than just our perception.

---

[11] F. Benedetti, H. S. Mayberg, T. D. Wager, C. S. Stohler, J. K. Zubieta, "Neurobiological mechanisms of the placebo effect," *J. Neurosci.* 25, no. 45 (2005): 10390–402.

[12] M. A. Flaten, T. Simonsen, H. Olsen, "Drug-related information generates placebo and nocebo responses that modify the drug response," *Psychosom Med.* 61, no. 2 (1999): 250–5.

[13] Irving Kirsch, "Specifying non-specifics: Psychological mechanism of the placebo effect," In A. Harrington, *The Placebo Effect: An Interdisciplinary Exploration* (Cambridge MA: Harvard University Press, 1997), 166–86.

The new paradigm outlined here would acknowledge the reality of the placebo effect. It would make it part of the "positive heuristics" of a research program instructing us which paths of research to pursue—instead of the negative heuristics of which paths to avoid. This changes placebos from a nuisance into a blessing. It would arguably keep placebos as biologically inactive, but at least active in many other ways that eventually may result in a biological outcome. It relates the placebo effect to the perception and expectation that the patient has "in mind"; if the substance is viewed as helpful, it can heal, but if it is viewed as harmful, it can cause negative effects— known as the *nocebo* effect.

One study found that for postoperative dental pain following the extraction of the third molar, a saline injection while telling the patient it was a powerful painkiller was as potent as a 6–8 mg dose of morphine.[14] Placebo effects can even last for a long time: over eight weeks for panic disorder, six months for angina pectoris, and two and half years for rheumatoid arthritis. To put it briefly, just *thinking* you are being treated can make you feel better, even for a long time.

There is already a lot of research that would fit much better in the new paradigm than the old one. Expectancy effects have been found to occur with a wide range of substances. In 1985, Irving Kirsch hypothesized that placebo effects are produced by the self-fulfilling effects of response expectancies in which the belief that one will feel different leads a person to actually feel different.[15] According to this theory, the belief that one has received an active treatment can produce the subjective changes thought to be produced by the real treatment. Another factor increasing the effectiveness of placebos is the degree to which a person attends to his or her symptoms— the so-called "somatic focus."

It will be the new paradigm that opens up research for the power of the mind. The study of placebos indicates that the mind and its sometimes unconscious effects are incredibly powerful instruments in treatment, and that we are getting but half the story in focusing so

---

[14] J. D. Levine, N. C. Gordon, R. Smith, H. L. Fields, "Analgesic responses to morphine and placebo in individuals with postoperative pain," *Pain* 10, no. 3 (1981): 379–89.

[15] Irving Kirsch, "Response Expectancy as a Determinant of Experience and Behavior," *American Psychologist* 40, no. 11 (1985): 1189–1202.

relentlessly on chemistry, biology, and genes alone. The effects of belief on human experience and behavior provide an entry point for a different kind of intervention. The process of administering placebos, along with the hopefulness and encouragement provided by the experimenter or doctor, affect the mood, expectations, and beliefs of the subject, which in turn may trigger physical changes such as the release of endorphins, catecholamines, cortisol, or adrenaline. The placebo effect triggers a self-healing effect based on the belief that a "fake" medication or a "fake" treatment is the "real" thing. This effect of the mind is so powerful that scientists actually have to adjust their experiments to compensate for it.

These effects are different from what the old paradigm would assert. In the old paradigm, there is sometimes a discussion of "top-down" processes. It has been said, for instance, that functional imaging upon placebo painkillers shows that the placebo response is mediated by "top-down" processes dependent on frontal cortical areas that generate and maintain cognitive expectancies based on dopaminergic reward pathways. As a consequence, diseases lacking major "top-down" or cortically based regulation may be less prone to placebo-related improvement.

However, the "top-down" approach of the old paradigm is very different from the "top-down" approach of the new paradigm. The "top" entity of the former is the *brain* with its different cortical areas, whereas the "top" entity of the latter is the *mind* with its thoughts and beliefs. Once we allow for the power of the mind in the new paradigm, people regain the power of self-healing. People who accept that the power of their beliefs can change reality are blessed with an incredible tool. Understanding this power creates the possibility of achieving your innermost desires—as well as fulfilling your negative prophecies. As the saying goes, "Whether you believe you can or can't, you're probably right."

One might even go one step farther by hypothesizing that placebo effects account for a major proportion of the positive effects of drugs. It has been shown that the placebo response is highly correlated to the drug response. Instead of administering "active" drugs, with side effects, one could opt for "inactive" placebos that use the power of the mind instead. The technique of hypnotic suggestion makes a case in point; it is explicitly intended to make use of the placebo effect by openly making use of suggestion and employing methods to amplify its effects.

There is, of course, the question of ethics. It may very well be unethical to use a placebo instead of using the "real" drug, but that holds only when seen from the old paradigm where everything centers around "the real thing." Withholding an effective drug by administering a placebo would then be unethical. However, we have a seeming paradox here, called the "Placebo Paradox": Once we acknowledge that placebos do have a healing effect in the new paradigm, it may also be unethical to withhold something that does heal—the placebo.[16] As long as the one administering the placebo is honest, open, and believes in its potential healing power, one could be ethically entitled to use the placebo effect.

In the above topics I discuss features that suggest that the new paradigm should be seriously considered. However, as the history of science shows, there is great resistance to paradigm shifts. Sometimes it takes decades for theories based on a new paradigm to gain a stronghold in the minds of other scientists. Examples can be found throughout the history of science. William Harvey never saw his theory of closed blood circulation fully accepted. Isaac Newton's gravitation theory required some eighty years before it was universally adopted. Alfred Wegener's theory of continental drift was embraced only fifty years later, after the acceptance of the theory of plate tectonics. For almost thirty-five years, Gregor Mendel's findings escaped notice. It took decades for antiseptics—discovered by Ignaz Semmelweis in 1847, by Louis Pasteur in 1862, and by Joseph Lister in 1867—to become generally accepted in surgery. Einstein's 1905 work on relativity remained controversial for many years, but later was adopted by leading physicists, beginning with Max Planck. This list could go on and on.

What about neuroscience—is it ready for a new paradigm? I maintain that the answer to the question "What makes you tick?" calls for an invisible mind, in addition to a visible brain. However, it will require a fundamental change in the old paradigm for neuroscientists to acknowledge this. Thomas Kuhn, who coined the

---

[16] David H. Newman, *Hippocrates' Shadow* (New York: Scribner, 2009).

term paradigm, spoke in terms of scientific revolutions. But he also used a quote from Max Planck:

> A new scientific truth does not triumph by convincing its opponents and making them see the light, but rather because its opponents eventually die, and a new generation grows up that is familiar with it.[17]

This statement is rather cynical and I would like to be more optimistic about the future of this new paradigm for neuroscience. But I must admit that most of the history of science is not on my side.

What makes it so difficult to change a paradigm? Well, first of all, individual scientists acquire knowledge of a paradigm through their scientific education. That is how they learn their standards, by solving "standard" problems, performing "standard" experiments, and eventually by doing research under a supervisor already skilled within the paradigm. Aspiring scientists gradually become acquainted with the methods, the techniques, and the presuppositions of that particular paradigm. Because of their training, scientists are typically unable to articulate the precise nature of the paradigm in which they work until the need arises to become aware of the general laws, metaphysical assumptions, and methodological principles involved in their paradigm.[18] My hope is that this book, in raising questions about laws and methods has created such a need, so we can find out what it is that really makes you "tick."

---

[17] Thomas Kuhn, *The Structure of Scientific Revolutions* (Chicago: University of Chicago Press, 1970). See particularly page 150.

[18] This is what Michael Polanyi called "tacit knowledge" in his books *Personal Knowledge* (London: Routledge, 1973) and *Knowing and Being* (London, Routledge, 1969).

Index

U

W

V